The Devil's Little Black Book

Regression Hypnotherapist's Troubleshooting Guide with Tips, Tricks & Even Scripts to Tweak Your Therapeutic Technique

Wendie Webber

The Devil's Little Black Book: *Regression Hypnotherapist's Troubleshooting Guide with Tips, Tricks & Even Scripts to Tweak Your Therapeutic Technique*

Wendie Webber

Copyright © 2024 Wendie Webber
All Rights Reserved.

All rights reserved. No part of this publication may be reproduced, distributed, or transmitted in any form or by any means, including photocopying, recording, or other electronic or mechanical methods without the prior written permission from the author, except in the case of brief quotations embodied in critical reviews and certain non-commercial uses permitted by copyright law.

The information given in this book should not be treated as a substitute for professional medical advice; always consult a medical practitioner. Any use of information in this book is at the reader's discretion and risk. Neither the author nor the publisher can be held responsible for any loss, claim, or damage arising out of the use, or misuse, of the suggestions made, the failure to take medical advice, or for any material on third-party websites.

ISBN Print Book: 978-1-0688514-0-7

TABLE OF CONTENTS

TABLE OF CONTENTS i
WHY READ THIS BOOK? i
CHAPTER 1: GOT RESISTANCE? 1
CHAPTER 2: ARE YOU SET? 15
CHAPTER 3: GOT A BRIDGE? 53
CHAPTER 4: WHY HYPNOSIS? 67
CHAPTER 5: GOT A REAL REGRESSION? 81
CHAPTER 6: GOT A STRONG BRIDGE? 95
CHAPTER 7: GOT THE REAL PROBLEM? 111
CHAPTER 8: RESISTANCE RESOLVED? 135
CHAPTER 9: GOT EVERYTHING? 151
CHAPTER 10: INNER CHILD? 175
CHAPTER 11: TESTED & INTEGRATED? 201
CHAPTER 12: BIG HAIRY-SCARY EVENT? 223
CHAPTER 13: SPIRITUAL ISSUE? 255
CHAPTER 14: GOT FORGIVENESS? 269
CHAPTER 15: UNFORGIVEABLE? 285
CHAPTER 16: THE CORRIDOR METHOD 301
CHAPTER 17: LASTING RESULT? 319
CHAPTER 18: GOT THE SYSTEM? 337
CHAPTER 19: WHAT IF ? ? ? 345
FINAL THOUGHTS 403
GLOSSARY OF TERMS 407

The Devil's Therapy Series 419
Wendie Webber 420

WHY READ THIS BOOK?

There's a problem with our profession. Trainings focus primarily on techniques and protocols. Yes, you need them. They are, after all, the tools of our trade. And in the hands of a skilled practitioner, you can use them to dramatically change a person's life for the better. But they're only tools. It's up to you to learn how to use yours masterfully. I want to help you to do just that.

In **The Devil's Therapy**: *Hypnosis Practitioner's Essential Guide to Effective Regression Hypnotherapy*, I shared a step-by-step approach to guiding your clients through the three phases of regression hypnotherapy:

The first phase is the Set-Up phase. This is where you establish the therapeutic relationship and therapeutic contract, identify the resolution keys, and train your client to be an active participant in their own healing.

Phase 1: Steps

1. Intake Process
2. Educational Pre-Talk
3. Test Readiness for Regression

The second phase is the Transformation phase. This is where you conduct the core work of Regression to Cause including Bridging back, testing for the ISE, conducting the uncovering process, releasing emotional blocks, reparenting the Inner Child and reframing the causal event.

Phase 2: Steps

4. Regress and Release
5. Inner Child Work

The third and final phase is the Verification phase where you test the results and encourage a full integration of all changes. The final step, in achieving a complete healing with effortless permanence, is the forgiveness work. (It comes last for a reason.)

Phase 3: Steps

6. Test and Integrate
7. Forgiveness Work

Most of the time, your sessions will go like clockwork. Your client will follow instructions, enter a state of somnambulism, and regress into the event that is responsible for generating unwanted symptoms. You'll guide the client to review, re-evaluate, and resolve the painful emotions trapped in that event. As a result, they'll gain insight into the cause of their problem, and emerge from the session feeling enormously better. But not always.

Sometimes, your session will go completely sideways. Most hypnosis schools don't teach this, but the *real* work of regression hypnotherapy is resolving client-resistance. Clients can be resistant to entering a state of hypnosis. They can be resistant to following instructions or allowing uncomfortable emotions to come to awareness. They can be resistant to facing painful events from the past. Resistance is simply fear, fear is an emotion, and emotions and feelings come from the subconscious mind. That's where you work.

> *The two questions I always ask myself are 'What if' and 'Why not?'* ~ **Jennifer Nettles**

Where **The Devil's Therapy**[1] answers the most important question, "Why do we do what we do when we do it?" **The Devil's Little Black Book** answers the question, "What if?"

> What if the client doesn't believe he was hypnotized?
>
> What if the client won't go into hypnosis?
>
> What if the client can't find a feeling?
>
> What if the client has an abreaction?
>
> What if . . .?

In this companion guide to **The Devil's Therapy**, I'm going to show you how to work around some of the more predictable ways resistance can rear its ugly head in a session. **The Devil's Little Black Book** will give you the pro tips and techniques you've been waiting for.

In Chapter 1, we're going to look at client resistance and what to do when sh*t happens in your sessions. We'll explore the five essential tools of regression hypnotherapy and how to tweak your technique when it comes to delivering suggestions.

---

[1] In my first book, I use a Grimm's Fairy Tale to illustrate a systemic approach to regression hypnotherapy comprised of seven steps.

In Chapter 2, we're going to dive into Phase 1 of the therapeutic process and how you can set your clients (and yourself) up to be more successful. We'll look at how many of the techniques you learned in basic training can be used as both preliminary and polishing techniques. You'll learn preliminary testing techniques, preliminary regression strategies, preliminary uncovering exercises, and how to use your first session wrap up to set up for the next session.

In Chapter 3, you'll learn the three steps to finding an effective Bridge to regress on, and what to do when the client has an abreaction or can't find or feel a feeling.

In Chapter 4, you'll learn strategies you can use to tweak the Elman induction, including a troubleshooting guide for each step in the process.

In Chapter 5, you'll learn how to get a real regression. We'll look at some of the problems that can occur during the induction process. You'll learn an effective test for somnambulism, and tips on how to deepen effectively.

In Chapter 6, you'll learn a six-step process to get a strong Bridge to regress on. You'll learn the Lily Pad approach to regression, and troubleshooting tips for when a client won't regress, loses the Bridge, or just doesn't want to "go there."

In Chapter 7, we'll dig into the uncovering procedure, how to identify the real problem using a 9-step process, and how to deal with the client's resistance to allowing uncomfortable feelings and memories to come to awareness.

In Chapter 8, we'll look at how to get rid of the more common types of resistance, such as vague responses, inability to see what's happening, feeling stuck, or abreacting.

In Chapter 9, we'll look at emotional releasing and how to ensure a lasting result using a five-step process. We'll look at when to regress or release, how to get more detail, and what to do when the client doesn't seem to be releasing the emotion.

Chapter 10 is all the core work of regression hypnotherapy – Inner Child Work. Here you will learn a seven-step process to transforming the Inner Child, including a troubleshooting guide for dealing with the thoughts and feelings of the Child. We'll also look at time-management strategies for when you're short on session time.

In Chapter 11, we'll look at testing and integrating techniques, including how to test to make sure the ISE is clear, and how to clear residual and secondary aspects. Included are techniques for framing, generalizing change, and generating insights.

You'll learn how to use Pro-Regression, the Grey Room Technique, and other methods to test and reinforce positive changes.

In Chapter 12, we'll look at how to deal with a big hairy-scary event. Included is a seven-step process, troubleshooting guidelines, and two client cases dealing with birth trauma and abuse.

In Chapter 13, we'll look at spiritual issues and what to do when a client goes to a past life. Included are client cases illustrating a stuck pattern from a past life and spirit attachment.

In Chapter 14, we'll look at how forgiveness is the healing, and the four steps to getting a complete resolution of the client's issue. Troubleshooting includes forgiving the Child, growing the Child up, testing and integrating, and keys to achieving complete forgiveness.

Chapter 15 focuses on what to do when the person who hurt the client is "unforgiveable." Included is a six-step protocol and three specific processes you can use when the client is holding onto a grievance.

In Chapter 16, you will learn how to use the Corridor method as a preliminary uncovering technique, regression technique, or forgiveness protocol. Included is an eleven-step stand-alone process, and post-forgiveness healing script.

In Chapters 17 and 18, we'll look at how to achieve lasting results using four testing techniques. We'll also look at how to conduct the preliminary check-in in subsequent sessions, how to use homework effectively, including a client case of intense anxiety, and how to be systematic using the three phases and four universal healing steps.

Chapter 19 contains a plethora of specific questions frequently asked by regression practitioners. This is where the rubber meets the road – in real sessions with real clients!

In addition, you'll find a glossary of terms in the back of the book.

Ready? Let's get started . . .

CHAPTER 1: GOT RESISTANCE?

Regression hypnotherapy is a journey of self-discovery that will take the client into uncharted territory. The client must be prepared to allow uncomfortable thoughts, feelings and memories to come to awareness. And many of the issues you'll work with will be rooted in unresolved, traumatic experiences from the past. Understandably, most people do not want to go there. But research shows that the only effective way to resolve a traumatic memory for good is to face the feelings trapped inside the memory. ~ **The Devil's Therapy**

When a client comes to you with a problem, it comes wrapped in a personal story. The conscious mind's story is the Pain Story. It tells you how the client is experiencing the pain of the problem. That's where they're stuck. The process of Regression to Cause will reveal the subconscious mind's story. This is an emotional story that begins at the Initial Sensitizing Event (ISE). It then develops through multiple Subsequent Sensitizing Events (SSEs).

Every client is going to be different because the territory of the mind is unique to each person. This means that, most of the time, you're guiding a client through unfamiliar territory. As a result, you're not always going to know what to do. There are two strategies that can help you to familiarize yourself with that territory. The first strategy is to experience the process of Regression to Cause hypnotherapy, yourself. Do your own work of self-healing. Know what you're asking your clients to do! The second strategy is to work with your dreams.

If you want a fun and easy way to get comfortable navigating the territory of the subconscious mind and feel fearless facilitating regression sessions, this is it. A dream is unadulterated, direct communication from the subconscious level of mind. For a hypnotherapist, that's *gold*!

Dream-working can help you to develop skills that are integral to facilitating effective regression hypnotherapy. For example, observation skills, uncovering skills, as well as Parts Work, which is central to inner child work and forgiveness work in regression hypnotherapy. Working with my own dreams has taught me how to listen to the subconscious mind and honor what it has to say. Through it, I learned how to translate the native language of the subconscious mind into terms the conscious mind can understand.

Client Resistance

While no two clients are ever exactly alike, they all share one thing in common: their subconscious mind is hardwired to protect them from any perceived threat. Each of us is naturally inclined toward a negative bias because it serves the subconscious mind's Prime Directive of survival. For example, if you ate the poison berries and they made you sick, you'll have the sense to avoid poison berries in the future!

Avoidance is always a big part of the client's presenting problem. Most people do not want to revisit painful events from the past. *Nobody* in their right mind wants to experience uncomfortable feelings and emotions! The conscious mind is resistant because it doesn't want to have to face unwanted feelings. It wants to avoid uncomfortable memories and emotions. The subconscious mind can be resistant because its Prime Directive is to protect the client from any perceived threat.

The problem is that, while avoidance strategies can help a person to cope with unwanted symptoms, they fail to get rid of the underlying problem. As a result, the symptoms tend to get worse over time. The truth is, you can't "make" a person heal, any more than you can "make" them relax. No script or protocol can address every eventuality. And you can't just do it *for* the client. The good news is that your *only* job is to identify and resolve the client's *resistance*. That's it. The client's resistance provides you with the information you need to guide the healing process effectively.

Resistance tells you where the client is being blocked from having, doing or being what they want. It also tells you when you're getting uncomfortably close to the very thing that is causing the client's symptoms. When you get dangerously close, sh*t can start to happen, often unexpectedly.

When Sh*t Happens

When sh*t happens during a session, and you don't know what to do, that's okay. Remain calm. If the client is losing their emotional sh*t, you losing *your* sh*t is only going to make things worse. This is because a person in an emotionally aroused state is in a state of hypnosis. Hypnosis is a hyper-aware state. If you're feeling afraid, your client is going to feel it. This will increase their resistance to allowing the feeling to be there.

When your session goes sideways, your Inner Critic will try to step in and take over. Don't let it. Thoughts such as "not enough . . . don't have what it takes . . . not perfect . . ." will only block your ability to stay present to the client. Give yourself the suggestion, "I've got this!" Remember, the subconscious mind is the emotional mind. Feelings and emotions are not bad or wrong. They're simply learned responses that have roots in the specific past experiences that caused them. The problem is that negative experiences generate uncomfortable feelings. Because experiences early in life shape identity, these unresolved emotional experiences become a part of a person's story about who they are, how life works, and what they deserve.

Recognize that the client is feeling out of control to an emotion. They're entering uncharted waters. Trust your internal guidance. It will provide a sense of safety in chaos. Get curious! Something interesting is happening. Say to yourself, "That's interesting . . ." Then, take charge of your session. Lean into it. Speak calmly and firmly and deliver suggestions to help restore a sense of safety to the client. That's what's most needed in that moment.

When sh*it goes completely sideways in a session, don't lose the lesson. Nobody has a 100% success rate. *Nobody*. When you fall on your face, get back up and learn from the experience by reviewing your session notes. If you keep good notes, you'll be able to identify when things started to go sideways. Then you can think about what you could have done differently. If you made some mistakes, forgive yourself. Give yourself permission to learn and grow from all your mistakes. Remind yourself that you are a work-in-progress – and you are becoming GREAT!

The Five Essential Tools

You really can transform a person's life with regression hypnotherapy. But it isn't merely another technique. It's a whole tool-suite of techniques and protocols that are designed to work together. *The Devil's Therapy* is a client-centered approach to facilitating regression hypnotherapy that uses the following five essential tools.

1. Regression to Cause
2. Parts Work
3. Uncovering Process
4. Forgiveness Work
5. Direct and Autosuggestion

The purpose of Regression to Cause therapeutic hypnosis is not merely to manage the client's symptoms. The goal is to realize a *lasting* result. To achieve this requires a systematic process of identifying and releasing the thoughts and emotions responsible for generating the client's uncomfortable symptoms. Developing your knowledge and skill utilizing these five tools will give you everything you need to transform lives for the better. Master these techniques and you'll feel confident working with practically any issue that comes through your office door.

Direct Suggestion

Suggestion is the basis of everything we do. Step back and look at your space through the eyes of a total stranger. What's your first impression? Because the subconscious mind's Prime Directive is safety, your session space needs to be a safe place for the client to be with you. It should instill confidence in the client.

Everything in your session room acts as a suggestion. Does it whisper "professional" or "amateur?" Is it neat and clean? Does it smell fresh? Does it provide adequate privacy? Is there a bathroom within proximity to your session room? Is your bathroom neat and clean? Anything that doesn't serve the healing process doesn't belong there. Clear out any distractions and get rid of the clutter.

Do you have pictures in your session room? Family photos might be appropriate for an executive office, but your healing space should be completely focused on meeting the needs of the client. Are your certificates framed professionally? A dollar-store frame hanging slightly askew doesn't say much about your value. Invest a few extra bucks in having your diplomas matted and framed. You're worth it.

Do you have plants and crystals in your session space? If your clients are metaphysical, there's nothing wrong with having a few crystals and gemstones around. But if you're running a general practice, make sure they're decorative and not demanding. If you keep plants, make sure they're vibrant and healthy. Dead or dying plants don't suggest positive outcomes. If you don't have a green thumb, consider silk plants. They don't require any upkeep and, these days, they look very lifelike.

What tools and resources do you need to facilitate the healing process effectively? Are they within easy reach when you're working with a client? For example, a blanket isn't just for warmth. It's a suggestion of comfort and safety.

If a client is wearing shorts or a short skirt, offering them a blanket provides a sense of security by allowing them to cover up. This ensures that they won't be distracted by feeling self-conscious or exposed. You can also offer a blanket to signal when the hypnosis is about to begin. Keep the blanket off to the side until you're ready to begin the induction process. When you pull it out and offer it to the client say, "Let's get comfy, shall we?" This anchors the blanket to the experience of going into hypnosis.

Regression hypnotherapy sessions are often a race against the clock. When you're seeing clients back-to-back, you need to keep your eye on the time to be on time for your next client. Also, if you want to use the time distortion test as a convincer, you'll need a big clock to ensure clients can see it without glasses. Place it somewhere obvious. That way, when the client emerges, they'll see it right away. Even if you're not doing a time distortion test, the client will often look at the clock and say, "Woah!" That's when you can say, "Time flies when you're in Lah-Lah Land …" You can then use this observation as a convincer by suggesting time distortion is a sign of the client's ability to be successful with hypnosis.

When you're just starting out, you need scripts and protocols. But you can't be observing your client's responses if you're reading a script. It's okay to use a script or a protocol while you're still learning. Having a cheat-sheet that you can reference during a session can act as a security blanket for *you*. It can help to keep you on task in sessions, which can help you to feel more confident and support you in getting more consistent results. But if the client thinks that you're reading a script, that thought will act as a suggestion that can bring your expertise into question. All it takes is a tiny seed of doubt to sabotage your success. Make sure your working papers are out of sight of your clients. Remember - out of sight is out of mind.

While simple issues respond well to suggestion alone, regression hypnotherapy is an interactive process that requires the client's participation. When you're working with an emotional issue, your primary job is always to work *with* the subconscious mind, not try to tell it what to do. This is a client-based approach to healing. You're not directly suggesting any change. Your suggestions are used to guide and support the client through the healing process. For example, to direct attention, amplify an emotion, encourage a deeper emotional release, validate an insight, etc. Based on what is revealed through the process, you can craft suggestions that are appropriate to the individual needs of the client.

While your ability to formulate and deliver clear suggestions will give you access to the memories and emotions at the root of the client's problem, your greatest asset during a regression hypnotherapy session is not your words. It's your ability to observe the client's responses to your suggestions. The subconscious mind communicates through feelings and emotions in the body. Feelings and emotions are experienced as physical sensations in the body. That's where your attention needs to be.

As the client talks about the problem, watch carefully for evidence of discomfort. Physical tightness or tension is evidence that something is rising from the subconscious level of mind to the surface of awareness. When that happens, bring the client's conscious attention to what's happening in the body. Affirm it by saying, "There's the feeling." Give it permission to be there.

Autosuggestion
Whether you're guiding a client through an induction process, deepening the hypnotic state, or utilizing a therapeutic technique, images and emotions are the language of the subconscious mind. You could be delivering direct suggestions or facilitating an autosuggestion process, but the most powerful suggestions evoke images and the feelings associated with them. Autosuggestion is where the client gives

themselves a suggestion. This technique was first developed by the famous French psychologist, Emile Coue, at the beginning of the 20th Century.

Coue recognized that suggestions don't last unless you reinforce them repeatedly. The purpose of compounding suggestions is to get targeted suggestions into the subconscious mind very powerfully where they will begin to take effect. Autosuggestion gives you a way to do this.

I used to wrap up every session with direct suggestions, but, over time, I came to prefer autosuggestion because regression hypnotherapy is not a passive process, and an engaged client doesn't have the opportunity to avoid feelings and memories. Autosuggestion is very effective at keeping the client's focus on feelings and emotions. You can use it to guide the client deeper into an uncomfortable feeling or to reinforce healing insights.

The way to use autosuggestion in your regression sessions is to, first, give your client a suggestion, then have them repeat it out loud. A direct suggestion followed by autosuggestion automatically has a compounding effect. This makes autosuggestion a highly effective amplification technique. For example, if the client is feeling an emotion of fear, you can increase the intensity of the emotion by instructing the client to repeat after you, "I feel scared!"

This is the quickest way to amplify any feeling because it's a statement of truth. Use it to amplify positive feelings such as calm, confidence, and well-being, or to acknowledge and reinforce positive changes that are occurring by validating new perceptions, healthier choices, or any shift toward a better feeling.

Affirmations vs Afformations

Would you rather be *told* to do something or *asked* if you are *able* to do it? A 2010 study revealed that, because of intrinsic human motivation, questions are more effective than positive affirmations. Professor Albarracin's [2] research into the motivating power of self-talk was published in the April 2010 issue of *Psychological Science Journal*.

The question she and her team of researchers sought to answer was which is more effective – a basic affirmation or a question?

In the first of two tests, 50 participants were asked to solve a series of anagram puzzles (rearranging letters within words to form new words, like when/hewn). Some of the participants were directed to tell themselves, "I will solve the anagram" while others were told to ask themselves, "Will I solve the anagram?" They were instructed to think of either the question or statement for one full minute before beginning the puzzle. The results? It turns out that asking a question outperformed the traditional affirmation *by over 85%*.

When a positive suggestion conflicts with a person's well-established beliefs and values, the protective function of the mind, or critical faculty, will ensure that the suggestion doesn't get in. Worse, some affirmations can make a person feel worse. But when an empowering *question* is offered, it magically slips past the critical faculty of the mind. Why? Because finding answers to questions is a function of the subconscious mind.

---

[2] Albarracin, Dolores and Ibrahim Senay, *Interrogative Self-Talk and Intention: Motivation Goal-Directed Behavior through Introspective Self-Talk: The Role of Interrogative Form of Simple Future Tense.* "Psychological Science. April 2010. Vol 21, Number 4.

"When a suggestion gets rejected, there will be no change." ~ **Gerald Kein, Omni-Hypnosis**

When we ask ourselves a question, the subconscious mind *automatically* goes looking for an answer. You can use this to bypass the critical faculty's defense system. The Law of Attraction states that what we focus on we tend to get more of. The problem is that human beings have a negative bias. As a result, the questions we ask ourselves tend to be negative and habitual. For example: "Why do I always screw up?" "Why me???" "Why do I keep blowing my diet?" "Why am I always late?" "Why don't people like me?" "How could I be so stupid?"

When you ask the subconscious mind a negative question, it will come up with all the reasons that suggestion is true. It goes to work finding all the "because's" to support that idea. This satisfies the conscious mind's need for reason and logic. The problem is that every 'because" becomes a subconscious motivation to achieve a specific outcome. As a result, habituated negative questions serve to reinforce a negative bias and can soon become self-fulfilling prophecies.

Human beings habitually ask questions. We do it consciously and unconsciously. Why not use it? Choosing better questions will allow the subconscious mind to do what it naturally does while encouraging it to come up with better answers. Noah St. John[3] calls this clever alternative to affirmations "af*for*mations."

An afformation is essentially an affirmation in the form of a question. For example: "Why do I always do the right thing?" "Why is it so easy for me to maintain my ideal weight?" "Why am I always on time?"

---

[3] Noah St. John, *Permission to Succeed*, Healthy Communications, 1999

"Why do so many people appreciate me?" "Why do I love to walk every day?" When we ask, "Will I?" the subconscious mind tends to say, "Hell, yes!" When we ask, "Why?" the subconscious answers, "Because …" When we ask, "How?" the subconscious says, "Let me count the ways."

Regression to Cause

The objective of Regression to Cause hypnosis is to locate the event(s) responsible for *causing* the client's presenting problem. This allows you to resolve the problem where it got started. The process of resolving the client's issue can employ a host of techniques, including preliminary uncovering techniques, amplification techniques, Bridging techniques, uncovering procedures, insight generating techniques, testing techniques and more. But the secret to achieving lasting results, working with real clients who are struggling with real problems, lies with the two Rs in Regression to Cause Hypnotherapy - "Regress" and "Release."

Regression is the process of going back to review events from the past. It's not merely an exercise in imagination. It is a process of accessing memories that are, to some degree, repressed. Often, these events are found in the client's childhood. Real regression involves revivification of the event. To achieve this requires a state of somnambulism.

Releasing is a powerful healing technique that, when coupled with regression, allows the discharge of painful emotions that have been trapped in past events. This is why regression hypnotherapy is sometimes called Abreactive Regression Therapy (ART). The hypnotherapist purposefully provokes an emotional response as a means of accessing a Bridge to past events.

Spontaneous regression is not uncommon in sessions and is invited as a welcome part of the healing process. In fact, abreactions often precede a spontaneous regression and are encouraged and utilized to resolve the client's issue. Provoking, amplifying, regressing, and releasing painful emotions requires quick reflexes. Sometimes you must work quickly to stay ahead of the resistance coming from both the conscious mind and subconscious mind.

Parts Work

Parts Work[4] is essential to effective regression hypnosis and forms the core work of the Transformation Phase of **The Devil's Therapy**. Most of the issues you're going to deal with in hypnosis will have their roots in childhood. This is because our core Parts are shaped by events very early in life – usually before the age of five. Our Parts express as thoughts, feelings, behaviors, and physical symptoms.

We have many Parts but the three primary Parts we work with in regression sessions are the Inner Child Part, the Adult/Grownup Part, and the Parent and/or Offender Parts of the client.

Uncovering Process

The purpose of the uncovering process is to identify and transform internal blocks to restore a sense of power to the client. The internal resources needed to heal already exist within the client, but they may be suppressed. Through the healing process, the blocks must be identified and released to gain access to internal sources of empowerment. For example, Parts that have been contributing to the presenting issue, once uncovered, can be transformed into positive capabilities. New capabilities can also be found in the past and brought

---

[4] Book recommendation: The Satir Model: Family Therapy and Beyond by Virginoa Satir, John Banmen, Jane Gerber and Maria Gomori

forward into the client's present life. Old capabilities can be revised and converted into new resources to empower the client in their daily life. As these resources are consciously identified, and reclaimed by the client, they can then be integrated fully.

Examples of uncovering and resourcing tools include a Sentence Stems Completion Exercise, the six basic uncovering questions of regression hypnotherapy, reframing, transferring positive resources from past experiences or through modeling, and insights generated through the healing process.

Forgiveness Work

Forgiveness opens the doors for healing to happen – physically, mentally, emotionally, and spiritually. You probably weren't taught this, but forgiveness isn't something we do. Forgiveness is something that happens through the process of releasing trapped thoughts and emotional energies. When the client lets go of the emotional charge, there's nothing left to generate unwanted symptoms.

Forgiveness happens the moment the client lets go of *the problem*. In **The Devil's Therapy**, forgiveness *is* "the healing." It happens the moment the client realizes that they've been doing it to themselves. They recognize that, subconsciously, they've been holding onto the problem, often for some very good reasons, but now they are free choose differently. They can hold onto the problem, or they can let it go.

CHAPTER 2: ARE YOU SET?

While you're interacting with the conscious mind, the subconscious mind isn't off somewhere else. It's right there sitting quietly off to the side, observing you, and deciding whether you can be trusted. The subconscious mind is duty-bound to protect the client. Safety is its Prime Directive. It will protect the client from any perceived threat – real or imagined. If you fail to win the trust of the subconscious mind, it will protect the client by blocking you. ~ **The Devil's Therapy**

Every hypnotherapist is schooled in the dual-mind theory, which states that we have a conscious mind and a subconscious mind. The conscious mind is where most people live - the thinking mind. We also have a subconscious mind. This part of us is working behind the scenes 24/7, primarily to protect us and keep us safe. The subconscious mind holds the key to the client's healing. But, to gain access to this information, the client needs to feel safe enough to let you guide the process. This is because the subconscious mind's primary concern is protecting the client from harm. It will protect the client from any perceived threat, real or imagined, including *you*. You need to make it safe for the client to follow your instructions.

The subconscious mind is the emotional mind, which learns through association and keeps a record of our past experiences for future reference. What makes any experience memorable is how it feels. Comfortable feelings and emotions are associated with happy memories. Uncomfortable feelings and emotions are associated with stressful experiences in the past.

Regression happens very naturally, given the right conditions. You just need to create the conditions where the client will allow it to happen. Because the subconscious mind learns through association, it naturally associates feelings with events from the past. The easiest way to encourage this to happen is to focus on the feeling that has everything to do with the client's presenting issue. This gives you a Bridge you can follow right back into the event that caused it. But to find a Bridge, you first need to make it safe for the client to allow you to guide the process.

The client needs to feel safe enough to enter the state of hypnosis. They need to feel safe enough to allow uncomfortable feelings to come to awareness. They need to feel safe enough to go back into painful past events. To do that, you need to gain the cooperation of both their conscious and subconscious minds. This is the purpose of your intake process - to establish the Therapeutic Relationship.

Establish the Relationship

The process of establishing the therapeutic relationship begins long before you start the hypnotic induction. It begins with your first contact with a prospective client. Healing requires a relationship based on trust. Before you can proceed with a new client, you need to make sure they're the right client for you.

If there's one strategy that will increase your confidence and success rate, it's this - *qualify your clients*. The purpose of your first contact with a prospective client is not to try to sell them a session. It's to qualify that they're the right client for you, and that you're the right therapist for them. The truth is you cannot be all things to all people. Why would you even want to be? Qualifying your clients will put you in the driver's seat of your sessions and improve your outcomes dramatically.

Once you have a qualified client, the next step is to conduct the intake process. Your intake[5] is a preliminary uncovering procedure which, if used strategically, allows you to gather the information you need to guide the healing process effectively.

Realize the client's conscious mind and the subconscious mind both have the power to block you. Taking a history of the client's problem helps to satisfy the conscious mind's need to feel heard and understood. It also gives you the opportunity to demonstrate to their subconscious mind that you can be trusted with "sensitive information." Prove to the subconscious mind that it's safe to hand over the reins of control. Only then will it let you guide the process.

While you conduct the intake process, you can gather the information you need to deliver an educational pre-talk that speaks directly to the specific needs and concerns of your client. For example:

1. How is the issue expressing as symptoms?
2. How long has it been a problem? When did it get started?
3. Is there a specific symptom pattern?
4. What emotions are connected to the problem?

---

[5] Learn more in *Ditch the Script: Get Everything You Need from the Client for Successful Hypnotherapy and Set Up to Wrap Up with Results*

5. Who is connected to the problem?
6. What is the client's therapeutic goal?
7. What specific conditions might support the client in achieving their goal?

As the client talks about the problem, pay close attention to information that triggers them emotionally. What do they think is the cause of the problem? Is there someone to blame? If so, what are their thoughts on forgiveness? Gently probing the specifics gives you the information you need to craft your pre-talk.

Your pre-talk is an important step in providing the safety needed by allaying irrational fears and instilling confidence in the process. All healing is self-healing. But it can take time for a person to feel safe enough to allow healing to happen. Your pre-talk allows your client to make an informed decision to let you guide the process. That's huge!

Establish the Contract

The educational pre-talk[6] for regression hypnotherapy is a preliminary uncovering technique that serves the purpose of establishing a therapeutic contract specific to Regression to Cause. This contract gives you permission to (a) induce hypnosis and (b) guide the client into painful past events that are contributing to the presenting issue. The client needs to understand the goal of regression hypnotherapy which is to find the event responsible for seeding the client's presenting issue, and to release the trapped emotions responsible for generating symptoms.

---

[6] Learn more in *Radical Healing: Hypnosis Practitioner's Guide to Harnessing the Healing Power of the Educational Pre-Talk*

Releasing emotions that got trapped in painful past events will result in healing. But for this to happen, you need the client's cooperation. The client must be willing to allow uncomfortable feelings and emotions to be part of the process. This will only happen with their consent.

What the client needs to understand is that their subconscious mind is not the enemy. The subconscious mind is the emotional mind. Its primary concern is to meet important needs, such as survival. That's good! To accomplish this, the subconscious mind keeps a record of past experiences for future reference. Comfortable feelings and emotions are associated with happy memories. Uncomfortable feelings and emotions are associated with stressful experiences in the past. This is how the subconscious mind learns - through association. As a result, it naturally associates to situations and events from the past.

Your job is to guide the process. The client's job is to do the work necessary to achieve their therapeutic goal by following your instructions. In other words, you are responsible for ensuring the client's safety while the client is responsible for the results. That's the Contract.

Prepare the Client

Not every client is going to be push-button ready for regression. You need to prepare them for the process. Regression hypnotherapy is an exposure therapy that brings to light the underlying cause of the client's issue. Once brought to conscious awareness, it can be released. The problem is that most people have been conditioned to avoid uncomfortable feelings. Not only does this make the subconscious mind a living hell, it generates resistance to "going there."

I'm not an advocate for dumping clients into their stuff in the first session. I want to establish safety by making the client's first session a positive experience. For this reason, I prefer to use relaxation hypnosis in the first session, whenever possible. This provides the ideal conditions for teaching a client how to work with you.

Preparing your client for regression hypnotherapy begins with teaching them how to enter the state of somnambulism. Somnambulism is a deeper state of hypnosis which allows the client to step into an event from the past and revivify the experience. They're not imagining, thinking about, or remembering. They're *feeling* the event as it was recorded by their subconscious mind. This gives you access to the hidden aspects that are calling for resolution.

Many of the techniques that you learned in basic hypnosis certification can be used effectively with regression hypnotherapy as both preliminary and polishing techniques. For example, self-hypnosis, direct and autosuggestion, guided imagery and ego-strengthening techniques are often used as stand-alone protocols for working with surface issues such as study-skills, sports improvement, and stress management.

Where these techniques really shine is when you're working with deeper issues. For example, direct suggestion, guided imagery, and Parts Work can be used as preliminary techniques to prepare the client for the deeper work of regression hypnotherapy. A hypermnesia exercise, positive regression and future pacing can be used for the purpose of ego-strengthening or to increase motivation. Tapping can be used to instill positive mental expectancy by providing proof that change is possible. Preliminary uncovering techniques such as Sentence Stems Completion Exercise or Color Diagnostics can also be used to identify specific aspects of the client's issue. You can use dream re-entry to uncover patterns and themes, triggers, grievances toward others, and resistance to facing certain issues or feelings that are contributing to the client's presenting issue. This information can help you to guide the regression process more effectively.

Preliminary Testing Techniques

Acceptability Testing

Autosuggestion is a very useful technique that can be used to get direct feedback from the subconscious mind. This can provide critical information to help and guide you in facilitating the healing process. You can use it to test the acceptability of a suggestion before you offer the suggestion!

When used as a testing technique, autosuggestion helps to keep the client tuned into the wisdom of the body. If a suggestion doesn't feel true, the client will feel it. This tells you that their subconscious mind is rejecting the suggestion. Repeating an unacceptable suggestion will only make the client's problem worse.

Whenever you offer a suggestion, there's going to be a response. When a suggestion is acceptable, the body will relax, and the client will feel sensations of comfort. Repeating an acceptable suggestion will increase the client's suggestibility to the concept or idea, thus compounding the power of the suggestion. But just because a suggestion sounds good to *you* does not mean that it is acceptable to the client's subconscious mind. Remember, the subconscious mind communicates with the conscious mind through feelings and sensations in the body. Whenever something happens, the subconscious mind generates a signal to let us know how safe we are. This signal takes the form of comfortable and uncomfortable feelings.

When the suggestion is *not* acceptable, the subconscious mind will let the conscious mind know by generating pressure or tension in the body. Tension doesn't feel good. It feels uncomfortable. That's resistance. Resistance tells you that there's a block to the suggestion. The subconscious mind is clearly communicating that what you are suggesting is not allowed. For some reason, your suggestion is "not okay" or "not true." This is useful information! When there's a block to a suggestion, the next step in the client's healing process is to release it. For example, "The thought (rejected suggestion) makes me feel (scared) in my (gut)."

To test the acceptability of a suggestion, give the client a suggestion to repeat out loud with instructions to notice how it feels in the body as she says it. Does it feel comfortable or uncomfortable? Where in the body does she feel "that" feeling? If it's a good feeling, you're good to go! Increasing focus on the sensations in the body will amplify awareness of "that feeling." Repeating the suggestion will compound the effect. As a result, the client will feel better and better. Bring this effect to the client's attention!

If the response to the suggestion is an uncomfortable feeling, ask the client to describe "that feeling." For example, if it had a color, what color might it be? If it had a shape, what might that shape be? If it had a size, a temperature, a vibrational quality, what might they be? If "that feeling" could speak, what would it say?

This last question can bring a Part forward. Giving the Part permission to speak can help you to identify what the specific objection to the suggestion might be. You can then decide whether to continue with Parts Therapy Work or bring up the emotion associated with that Part and Bridge back to the event that caused that Part to form.

Muscle Response Testing

Subconsciously held beliefs that conflict with the conscious mind's wishes can be uncovered through muscle testing. You can also use it to provide evidence that what a client *thinks* and how they *feel* are not always in alignment. For example, I used Muscle Response Testing (MRT) to uncover a critical block to a cancer client's ability to heal. When I tested the client on the statement, "I want to live," the statement tested as "true." I then tested the opposite statement, "I want to die." This statement *also* tested true, much to the surprise of the client. This realization proved to be a pivotal moment in this client's healing process.

If you're not trained in kinesiology or MRT you can still teach the client to pay attention to the wisdom of the body. Because feelings and sensations in the body are how the subconscious mind communicates with the conscious mind, teaching your clients to pay attention to the wisdom of the body can help you to get better results during regression sessions. You can also use MRT as a preliminary technique to provide proof to a client that their body is the subconscious mind. For example, Emotional Freedom Technique (EFT) utilizes MRT to show the client how the body knows the truth using the following two steps:

First, ask the client to make a statement they know to be true. For example, "My name is (Client Name)." Then gently test the muscle strength in response to the statement. This establishes a baseline for truth.

Second, ask your client to make a statement that is obviously a lie. For example, "My name is (Meryl Streep/Donald Duck)." Muscle test on this statement. This demonstrates how the body knows what is true and what is not true.

Ideomotor Signaling

While you can use ideomotor signaling as a means of communicating with the subconscious mind, this limits you to yes/no questions which, as an uncovering procedure, is pretty clunky and time consuming. The subconscious mind is already communicating through feelings and sensations in the body. Why not use it?

Tapping Techniques

Tapping or Emotional Freedom Technique (EFT) is a form of psychological acupressure belonging to the field of Energy Psychology. According to its developer, Gary Craig, the cause of all negative emotions and pain is a disruption in the energy system of the body.

Tapping focuses on releasing trapped energies from the meridian system of the body to help balance energy flow to support health and healing. Regression hypnotherapy focuses on uncomfortable feelings in the body. Why not use tapping as a preliminary technique to get rid of resistance to feeling an uncomfortable feeling before you begin the process of regressing the client?

Not only will this make more of the feeling available to work with, teaching the client how to find, feel, and release an emotion will give you a better client to work with. First, use it as a preliminary technique to provide proof to the client that it's possible to feel better. Then use it to release trapped emotions in events from the past.

Don't know tapping?

If you don't yet know tapping, you can use autosuggestion. But tapping involves a ritual that has been shown to calm the amygdala (alarm system) of the brain. It's worth it to learn the basics. In the meantime, you can add a tapping element by inviting your client to tap on the Karate Chop point (the fleshy region on the side of the hand). This will help to increase focus, which will allow for a deeper release. The key is to maintain focus on the problem while tapping and talking. (This makes tapping a covert induction.) Tap gently – about the same pressure as drumming your fingers on the arm of your chair. The object is to stimulate the meridian points, not hammer in a statement/suggestion.

Alternatively, you can have the client rub the neuro-lymphatic release points on the chest. To find a neuro-lymphatic point, poke around on the upper chest region until you find a tender spot. The sore spots are located roughly in the area where you would slip your thumbs through your suspenders. Gently rub or tap on that spot while speaking the suggestion out loud. You can even have the client place a hand over each chakra on the front of the body. Six of the seven major chakras have been found to correspond to nerve plexuses in the body.

Formulating Set-Up Phrases

Releasing is part of the core work of regression hypnotherapy. It begins with teaching the client to accept their feelings. The traditional EFT set-up phrase uses a self-acceptance statement, "Even though I have this (problem), I accept myself."

You can adapt this statement to any issue. But the problem we want to target is a feeling inside that the client doesn't like. That's how they know there's a problem - it doesn't feel good. As a result, the client is resistant to allowing that feeling to come to awareness.

Teach the client that there's nothing wrong with feeling their feelings. Resistance to feeling a feeling is the client rejecting a Part of themselves. This only adds to their distress. Releasing gives that Part of them permission to express.

Step 1: Make the Feeling Acceptable

Start by focusing on making the feeling acceptable. You can do this by validating the truth of what the client is experiencing. Statements of validation increase rapport with both the conscious and subconscious minds because you're reinforcing what is already true. This makes it an acceptable suggestion. For example, "Even though I have this anxiety problem (true)/ and it doesn't feel good (true)/ this is *my* feeling (true) / and I'm allowed to feel it (transitional truth) / so I accept this feeling (the intended suggestion)."

Step 2: Find the Feeling in the Body

Once the client has given themselves permission to feel the feeling, you can ratchet up a notch by increasing the client's awareness of "that feeling" by bringing the client's attention to the body. Where do they feel that feeling in their body? Validate it! For example, "Even though I feel anxious, and I can feel it in my gut, this is *my* feeling, so I accept this feeling, and I deeply and completely accept myself." This is an amplification technique. It will make more of the feeling available for releasing.

When you're first teaching the client how to tap, keep it simple. It's okay to use whatever words the client uses, at first. This will validate the truth of what they're experiencing which will invite more of the feeling to bubble up to awareness. For example, if the client uses the word "anxiety", it's okay to start the tapping process on "anxiety."

Have the client tap on the Karate Chop point while repeating the setup phrase three times. Then, facilitate a round of tapping gently on each point on the body five or six times while repeating the reminder phrase. For example, "This fear." Or "This weight problem." Or "This fat."

Step 3: Name the Emotion
Once the client is focused on the feeling in the body, teach them how to name emotions. For example, "Give me another word for that anxious feeling in your gut." Or simply ask, "If that feeling in your gut was an emotion, what would it be?"

If you can guide the client to name an actual emotion such fear, sadness, or anger, you'll get a deeper release. Remember, it's all about finding and feeling the feeling. "That feeling" is an emotional signal coming out of the event that caused it. When the client can find, feel, and name an emotion, they'll hand you the Bridge to the ISE.

The secret to getting rapid results lies in grinding down to the specifics. The more specific you can be with your setup phrase, the better your result will be. For example, "Even though I have this fear in my tummy . . ." Or, "Even though I have this weight problem, and it makes me feel FAT, and the thought 'fat' makes me feel (sad, scared, angry, etc.) . . ."

Step 4: Make the Feeling Reasonable
When the client names an emotion, add a statement of commitment. For example, "I'm allowed to feel it and I'm allowed to release it."

Start by affirming everything that has been accepted, so far. For example, "Even though I *do* feel scared (truth)/ and I can feel it in my gut (truth) / this is *my* feeling (truth)" . . . Then add, "I'm allowed to feel it / and I'm allowed to release it / so I can feel better."

An alternate approach is to add a "because" statement to make it reasonable for the client to *have* "that feeling." For example, "Even though I have this scared feeling in my gut/ I don't have to feel scared for the rest of my life/ I'm allowed to feel it / and I'm allowed to release it/ *because* this is *my* feeling . . ."

Step 5: Add a Statement of Self-Acceptance
Complete each set up phrase with a statement of self-acceptance. For example, ". . . and even though I *have* this feeling /I deeply and completely accept myself."

This is a practice in self-acceptance. When the client makes a statement of self-acceptance despite *having* that feeling, they are accepting the Part of themselves that is responsible for generating "that feeling," whether it be fear, sadness, anger, or something else.

Affirming the subconscious "truth" increases rapport with the subconscious mind. Adding a statement of commitment – "I'm allowed" - gives the conscious mind what it most wants – a sense of control. Incorporating "because" statements such as "this is my feeling" or "so I can feel better" provides reasons for letting go of the uncomfortable feeling.

Step 6: Tap Through the Points
This set of suggestions gives you everything you need to tap through the points. The truth is that the client is allowed to feel it and they're allowed to release it to feel better. Let them prove this to themselves.

The reminder phrase could simply be "this feeling," but tapping on "this scared feeling in my gut" is much more specific and, therefore, much more powerful. As a result, it will yield a much quicker release and its corresponding sense of relief.

Because each meridian point corresponds to a specific feeling(s), when you're tapping a round, you can always choose to tap a little longer on the specific point that corresponds with the emotion the client is releasing. This may help to get a more complete release of the feeling. For example:

- **Eyebrow**: trauma, frustration, restlessness
- **Side Eye**: rage
- **Under Eye**: anxiety/fear, nervous, craving
- **Under Nose**: embarrassment
- **Chin**: shame
- **Collar Bone**: grief, anxiety, insecurity
- **Heart**: unhappiness
- **Top of Head**: clarity (use for confusion or to reinforce a moment of insight)
- **Thumb**: intolerance, arrogance
- **Index Finger**: guilt
- **Middle Finger**: jealousy, addictive cravings
- **Little Finger**: anger
- **Karate Chop**: sadness, reversals

Work with whatever the client gives you. Then, add something to it. Find the feeling in the body. Accept it. Name the emotion. Accept it. Give it permission to be there. Then, release it.

Preliminary Regression Techniques

Most of the problems we deal with in regression hypnotherapy sessions have their roots in childhood. To get there, you need to bring up an uncomfortable feeling to Bridge back to specific event that caused the feeling. But most clients are resistant to allowing uncomfortable feelings to come to conscious awareness. You can bypass much of the resistance in the first session by using the following hypermnesia exercise.

Hypermnesia Exercise

Hypermnesia means "enhanced recall." It's not a real regression, but you can use it to prepare your clients for real regression. Instead of dumping the client into their stuff, why not prepare them for the journey? You can also use it to uncover resource states, facilitate ego-strengthening, and to teach your client how to work with you in a regression session. If the client is ready for regression, you'll find that the hypermnesia exercise can easily be converted into a real regression.

First, guide the client into hypnosis and deepen to state. Then, invite them to *remember* some positive events from childhood. The focus is on pleasant memories of feeling safe and secure. For example, almost everyone has pleasant memories from childhood of watching snow gently drifting down. It's quiet and peaceful, safe and secure.

Not only does this make a delicious deepening technique, it acts as a natural segue into recalling other pleasant memories from childhood. For example: "And just like the way snow falls .... and every gentle flake of snow … comes down so slowly and so peacefully … you can allow your thoughts to just drift, drift … to a deeper level of rest … wrapping the trees and the ground in a soft blanket of quiet comfort ……. so peaceful and so safe … And the longer you watch the flakes coming down, down, down … the more relaxed you become… sinking down to a more positive way of thinking, feeling, and behaving, at that automatic, unconscious level …"

Following this pleasant memory deepening technique, you can invite the client to recall a pleasant memory of being in or around water. Everyone has experienced being in or around water as a child. For example, a puddle, or a pond, or even bath time, but a happy, pleasant memory of being in or around water. Instruct the client to let you know when they find that pleasant memory. Then, when the client indicates that they have found it, help them to associate more fully into the scene.

As they reconnect with the positive feelings and emotions associated with the memory, they are accessing resource states that can be directed for the purposes of ego-strengthening. It's all in them now. Just don't rush the process. You're teaching the client how to revivify an event within the context of a safe environment. This gets rid of the resistance and gives the client a transferable skill by teaching them how to work with you in regression sessions.

Guide the client to step into the scene by using the basic uncovering process. This makes the uncovering process familiar to the client and, therefore, safe. For example, "First impression . . . does it feel like it's daytime or nighttime? Does it seem like you're inside or outside? Are you alone or with someone? Who are you with? Where are you? What's happening? How does that make you feel?"

The first three uncovering questions help to increase the client's focus of attention, which deepens the hypnosis, while bringing more awareness of the details of the event to conscious awareness. Once you have fleshed out the scene, give the suggestion to, "Let all those good feelings (associated with that memory) come back to you now." Then, give the client a few moments to enjoy *just being there*. As the client soaks up the goodness, she is allowing herself to connect more deeply with her "good" feelings. Realize that healing is happening.

Remind the client, "You're allowed to let *all* your good feelings come back to you. These are *your* feelings." Then, give the suggestion to recall another positive experience. For example, being on or around a bicycle. It could be their bicycle, or a friend's bicycle, or any bicycle. Instruct the client to let you know when that happy memory comes to mind. Then, repeat the preliminary uncovering process to increase awareness of the scene and amplify the feelings associated with that memory. Once again, give the client a few moments to enjoy this resource state.

Make it a yummy experience! What you're doing is teaching your client that it's safe to allow feelings and memories to be a part of the process. Helping the client to reclaim these better feelings will give you a more resourceful client to work with when it comes time to dive into painful memories. It also reminds the client that her *good* feelings are still there, inside of her; she hasn't lost her ability to feel good. This can be a very emotional experience for some clients. There may be a few tears. Insights can arise.

Whatever comes to awareness, encourage the client to *let* herself feel the feeling fully. Then, when the client is ready, move onto another common childhood experience such as being on or around a swing. It might be the client's swing set. It could be a friend's swing set. It could be at a park or a school yard.

Again, instruct the client to let you know when that happy memory comes to mind. Repeat the preliminary uncovering procedure to deepen the emotional connection.

Find the memory and you'll find the feeling associated with that memory. Let all the good feelings come back to awareness. Give the client permission to fully enjoy the positive feelings and emotions associated with that experience. Then, reinforce the permission to allow those feelings. For example, "You're *allowed* to let all your good feelings come back to you." Or, "You're *allowed* to feel all your feelings." Or, "You're *allowed* to feel safe/comfortable/happy (or whatever the Child is experiencing.)"

Regression happens naturally under the right conditions. Because there's no resistance to experiencing happy childhood memories and emotions, this non-threatening approach can get you into the ballpark of the causal event, without triggering unnecessary resistance. Giving your client a yummy first experience of hypnosis with you removes resistance to "going there" in subsequent sessions. If you're lucky, you might even find the opportunity to convert the hypermnesia exercise into a full-blown regression session. Effortlessly[7].

Positive Regression

The hypermnesia exercise creates the right conditions for regression to happen very easily. Each time the client remembers a positive, happy event, they experience the enjoyment of being a Child. As this happens, the client is stepping into the experience *being* the Child. The deeper the client goes into the feelings associated with those childhood memories, the deeper they will go into hypnosis.

---

[7] Learn more in Ready for Regression: Hypnosis Practitioner's Guide to Preparing Clients for Effective Regression Hypnotherapy/

The deeper the hypnosis, the less they will be trying to remember, and the more they will be experiencing by revivifying the event. You can then convert this experience to a real regression, quite easily, because the client is already regressing. All you need to do is amplify all the good feelings, then offer the suggestion to, "Go to an earlier time where you're feeling this good, where you're just having fun."

Use a playful tone of voice as you suggest that it might be a celebration, like a birthday party. It might be their birthday party, or a friend's birthday party. It might be Christmas, or a special celebration. A happy time of celebrating and just having fun. When the client indicates that they have found the memory, repeat the uncovering procedure.

Give the client a few moments to enjoy the good feelings and reclaim the right to feel good. Then, reinforce their permission to allow feelings to be a part of the process.

If you have time, instruct the client to go to a time when she is feeling deeply relaxed. For example, 'Feeling so calm and so relaxed, so comfortable, peaceful and serene. It might be snuggled up all comfy and cozy . . . or a special place that you love . . . like a garden or in nature . . . it might be on vacation . . . or even RIGHT NOW. In fact, it might even be the FIRST TIME that you're feeling the wonderful, pleasant, comfortable feelings of being sooooo relaxed, and soooo at ease, that the only thing you care about is how deeply relaxed you feel. And as that feeling comes on, let me know."

Don't be surprised if the client goes right back into the womb! When that happens, you have a wonderful opportunity to plant a few seeds *before the ISE* happens.

If you're pressed for time, just give the client a few moments to enjoy this deeply relaxed state. For example, "That's right, go deeper relaxed, now. Just let yourself enjoy the simple pleasure of relaxing in this way. All is well. Allowing relaxation to flow through you, from the top of your head to the bottoms of your feet. Flowing wonderfully through every cell of your body, and throughout your nervous system. And notice what it's like to feel so safe, and so secure. Feels good, doesn't it? . . . That's right."

Preliminary Uncovering Exercises

The Stems Completion Exercise

Some clients do not respond well to direct questions. When a client interprets questions as a form of interrogation, your questioning will be perceived as a threat. If you ask too many direct questions, the client will shut down emotionally. That's just not helpful.

One of the most useful methods of getting answers is to use a Sentence Stem Completion Exercise or "Stems". A sentence stem is an open-ended question. To use it, you offer the client the beginning of a statement to repeat. You then invite the client to complete the sentence by putting an ending on it. For example, "My name is (put an ending on it.)"

Stems Completion Exercise is a valuable tool you can use to ensure that you are not creating false memories by leading the client. You simply offer an open-ended question. The client finishes the sentence. The answers always come directly from the client's own mind.

As an interactive process, Stems can help you to quickly identify specific aspects that are contributing to the client's issue. It also teaches the client to set aside thinking and focus on first impressions rather than trying to come up with the "right answer." This can help to prepare your clients for the uncovering process of regression hypnotherapy.

Stems Completion can be used to identify a Bridge to the past because, when you offer a fill-in-the-blank question, it forces the subconscious mind to associate to the cause of that specific feeling. This can bring up a strong emotion to Bridge back on. For example, invite the client to say, "I feel . . ." and put an ending on it. Then, locate that feeling in the body. Name the emotion behind that feeling and you have just identified a specific signal coming out of the Initial Sensitizing Event.

You can also use Stems Completion while in a past event to uncover the cause of the emotion you Bridged back on. For example, during the uncovering procedure, the Child reports that the Offender is looking at her in a way that makes her feel uncomfortable. Offering a Stem such as, "That look on his face makes me feel ... (put an ending on it)" helps you to connect the emotion to what's happening in the event. If the client says, "I feel scared" the next Stem to offer might be, "I feel scared *because* ... (put an ending on it)."

You can use "because" in a Stem to grind down through multiple layers of thoughts and feelings trapped in an event. For example, if the Child says, "I feel scared *because* Mommy is leaving me!", the next Stem to offer might be, "The *thought* 'Mommy is leaving me' makes me think . . . (put an ending on it)."

Feelings don't come out of nowhere. There is always a thought that precedes the feeling. *That* thought is the cause of *that* feeling. The feeling is never the problem. It's a response that forms an energetic signal transmitting from the event that caused it.

What happened in that event isn't the problem, either. The *real* problem has to do with how the ISE was being interpreted at the time it occurred, which has everything to do with the cognitive and emotional maturity of the client at the age the event happened.

The Child in a regression is the conscious mind at the age the client has regressed into. The conscious mind's job is to make sense of things. This provides a sense of control. But how an experience is being interpreted isn't always accurate, especially when the Child is feeling overwhelmed. Because these thoughts are recorded without critical thinking, they can become beliefs. That's the fundamental problem - thoughts become beliefs, and beliefs drive behavior and generate physical and emotional symptoms.

Follow the feeling to find the thought. The cause of "that feeling" is always going to be a specific thought. For example, if fear Bridges back to a frightened Child whose thought is, "I'm going to die!" you have just identified the thought-cause of "that fear". The next step is to instruct the Child to say, "The thought [I'm going to die] makes me feel [scared!]" This validates the subconscious truth – feeling scared - while teaching the conscious mind to make a distinction between thinking and feeling. That is the first step in putting the client back in control. To resolve that thought-feeling combo, reality-check the thought of the Child with adult consciousness. For example, "Grownup, (Child) thinks she's going to die . . . *Is that true?*"

If the thought is *not* true, this realization can discharge a tremendous amount of unnecessary emotional distress. It also helps the client to discover how her own thoughts are generating the problem while giving you a wonderful opportunity to reinforce these insights by compounding the newer, better "truth". For example, "Grownup must be telling you the truth because Grownup *is* you, all grown up. She came all the way back here to help you! Isn't that nice? Now you know! If she's still here, that means you're going to get through this. She's living proof that you get to grow up! How does *that* make you feel?"

The Color Diagnostic Technique

The Color Diagnostic Technique can be used as both a diagnostic tool and a polishing technique. As a diagnostic tool, it helps to enhance the client's body awareness, giving you a way to uncover negative imprints (stuck energy in the body-mind system). You can also use it to test for residual aspects. As a polishing technique, the Color Diagnostic Technique can be used to amplify positive thought and emotional energies once they have been established as acceptable.

Invite the client to go inside and do a scan of the body to get a general sense of how it feels. Good/bad? Comfortable/uncomfortable? If there's some discomfort present, focus on releasing "that feeling." If/when the body feels comfortable, proceed to the next step.

Instruct the client to imagine filling the body with color. Stephen Parkhill used orange light as a diagnostic technique. Cal Banyan uses white milky liquid to test for attachments. I found that pouring blue light in through the top of the head works very well. Alternatively, you can invite the client to sense or feel which color they need. Then, instruct them to imagine, sense and feel that color entering the body through the top of the head and filling it completely.

Here, you can enhance the experience by using a quick progressive relaxation patter. For example, "Imagine, sense, see, or feel that (blue) color entering the body through the top of your head. That's right.

Allowing that particular color blue to flow down into the head, into the front and the back, filling it completely. Allowing that blue to flow down the back of the neck and throat into the shoulders" etc.

Once the body is saturated with color, instruct the client to do a scan of the body, from the top of the head to the tips of the toes, and notice if there is any place the color didn't go.

If there is an area where the color *didn't* go, focus attention there and either (a) release the block to allow that quality of color, or (b) identify the Part that is expressing, name the emotion, and regress to an event in the past.

If the color was accepted throughout the body, pour in suggestions for positive change and anchor them to that color. For example, "From now on, whenever you see the color (blue), it reminds you . . ."

Dream Re-Entry

A dream is a subconscious experience. As a result, the subconscious makes no distinction between a daydream, a night dream, or "this" dream. All are experienced as valid realities. Because the subconscious mind makes no distinction between real and imagined, you can explore a night dream, create a daydream, or guide a person into a past event or an imagined future. After all, they all draw upon personal experiences stored at a subconscious level of mind that take the form of symbolic, internal representations that act as containers of personal meaning.

This is the basis of Parts Therapy Work.

Hypnotherapy naturally stirs up subconscious content which can result in your clients experiencing vivid dreams between sessions. When a client reports that they had a dream following a session, you have a wonderful opportunity to access pure, unadulterated subconscious information that can help you to find a Bridge for regression, identify and release trapped emotions, and/or test the results between sessions.

A dream is an emotional event. The more emotional the dream experience, the more "real" it is to the client. This is because the contents of a dream are based entirely on a person's history. The sensations and emotions evoked by a dream are real and have roots in the client's past. The client's subconscious mind knows why they're seeing you. As a result, "that feeling" will very likely be connected to the issue you're working on![8]

When a client presents a dream, treat it as you would a recent event. Invite the client to share with you what happened in that dream event. Then, induce hypnosis and guide the client to step into the dream scene and tell you the story from the beginning. Daytime or nighttime? Inside or outside? Alone or with someone? What's happening? The moment the client bumps into an uncomfortable feeling, you have a choice. You can use it to bring up a Bridge to the past, or simply release "that feeling."

The Echo Technique

The Echo Technique is a form of mindfulness meditation like the practice of Vipassana[9] or 7th Path Self-Hypnosis™[10]. You can use it as

---

[8] Dream Healing Practitioner Guidebook: *A Healer's Guide to Uncovering the Secret Messages of Your Dreams*
[9] Insight Meditation
[10] Calvin Banyan

a single-session stand-alone process, or as a preliminary technique to release some of the surface pressure before diving into the regression work.

The Echo Technique combines beautifully with tapping and auto-suggestion. This turns it into a covert and slightly confusional induction. The client will naturally enter a state of hypnosis which means you don't need to use a formal induction. This gives you a way to work with clients who aren't ready to "do hypnosis."

Where the Echo Technique truly shines, is when you use it as a polishing technique. At the end of a session, you can use it to (a) uncover and release residual aspects and (b) reinforce the positive changes that are occurring because of the session.

Once the client has learned the process, you can assign it as a homework assignment. This gives you a simple technique you can use with virtually anyone to get them working with their own internal guidance system.

Step 1: Formulate a Suggestion
If you're using The Echo Technique as a *preliminary technique*, treat it the same way you would a self-hypnosis training session. Formulate a suggestion that is relevant to the client's therapeutic goal or desired behavior. The more specific the suggestion is, the more effective it will be.

If the client has a big goal chunk down. What is one step toward the final outcome they desire?

To use The Echo Technique as a *polishing technique*, formulate a suggestion, based on the client's session, that reflects the new level of 'truth' or desired outcome. For example, if the client experienced a profound insight or a significant shift in some regard, you can turn it into a suggestion by using a statement of validation to reinforce the client's change in perception.

"I am ...." (self-image statement)

"I can ..." (self-confidence statement)

"I choose ..." (self-empowerment statement)

Step 2: Tap and Notice

Once you have formulated a suggestion, instruct the client to start tapping at the Eyebrow point while saying the formulated statement of truth. As the client says the suggestion out loud, remind him to stay focused inside and notice what comes up *in response* to the idea that is being suggested. It might come as a sensation in the body. It might be an emotion, or it might be a thought. It could be a picture or a memory. Remind the client that whatever comes up is okay - this is how the subconscious mind communicates. It speaks through feelings and emotions, pictures and memories. That's the 'echo'.

There's no need to do anything with the echo. Just let it come to conscious awareness. Let the client know that the moment something comes to awareness, to report it to you. That's it. Remind the client to set aside thinking, judging, or trying to make sense of things. The only thing the client needs to do is (a) notice the echo, (b) let you know when it comes. It doesn't take very long. The subconscious mind works quickly. The echo will come to the surface within two or three seconds.

The Echo Technique can easily be combined with other processes such as "Afformations". For example, "Why do I always LOVE practicing self-hypnosis?" (Echo, "No I don't.") Move to the next point and repeat the affirmation.

No echo?
The process will automatically bring up thoughts and feelings. If the client doesn't notice something right away, it's probably because the client is not paying close enough attention. Maybe his mind wandered off. That's okay. It's a practice, after all, not a "perfect". Instruct the client to repeat the suggestion and *focus more carefully inside*.

The 'echo' will come almost instantly. The trick is for the client to *notice* his first impression. This is an exercise in paying attention. The only thing we care about is the client's first sense. It might be a feeling or sensation in the body. It might be an emotion like fear or sadness. It might come as a picture, or a memory. Whatever comes, as soon as it comes to awareness, move on to the next tapping point, and repeat the statement.

Too many echoes?
Sometimes, two or three echoes can seem to come to awareness at the same time. They don't really. It's just that the subconscious mind works at lightning speed and the conscious mind can't keep up. If the client experiences a barrage of echoes at once, acknowledge the first echo, or the strongest echo, then move to the next point. The echo isn't what's important. What's important is the focus of attention.

Positive echo?
Internal beliefs that agree with the statement of "truth" will be experienced as a positive echo. When this happens, your client is in a

highly receptive state. Direct and auto-suggestion offered at this time can have a powerful transformative effect.

The goal is for all the echoes to be positive. When a positive echo comes to awareness, repeating the suggestion will have a compounding effect.

Negative echo?

Any objection to the suggestion will be brought to light through discomfort. That's resistance! Continuing to tap while repeating the suggestion will help to release the block.

If an objection is persistent, quantify the feeling using a Subjective Unit of Distress (SUD). On a scale of 1 to 10, where 10 is the strongest, how strong is that feeling? Tap a full round on that specific aspect. Then, take another SUD. The goal is to get that aspect down to zero.

Won't release?

If the objection won't release, switch to age regression and resolve the problem where it got started. Instruct the client to focus on "that feeling." Amplify it to ensure a strong Bridge and find out what happened to cause that feeling.

Short on time?

If you're short on time, wait until most of the echoes are positive before wrapping up your session. Then, assign The Echo Technique as a homework assignment between sessions. The more residual stuff the client releases between sessions, the less you'll have to deal with in session, and the quicker you'll achieve the results.

The Fork in the Road/Crossroads Technique

To get the results you're after, you need your clients to be highly motivated. Remember, not everyone is ready, willing, or able to begin the journey of regression hypnotherapy, especially if they're heavily invested in external solutions. The Fork in the Road or Crossroads Technique is traditionally used as an imagery exercise to assess and increase a client's motivation for change.

What you need to know is - how much of a problem is this for the client? How much pain is the client in? What factors are contributing to the problem? What situations or people act to trigger the problem? What specifically needs to change? Who is part of the problem? What are the consequences of failing to resolve the problem? How will the client know when they have truly resolved the problem?

It's difficult to identify these key elements with a guided imagery exercise. But when facilitated as an interactive process, the Fork in the Road Technique goes beyond merely exacerbating the pain of the problem to increase client motivation for change. You can use it to identify specific blocks and sources of empowerment to aid the client. That's valuable information!

Step 1: Establish a Path
To begin, establish a path. Behind the client lies the past. Before them lies the future. Give the suggestion that the client has come to a crossroads, and to now notice how the path they've been on forks to the left and to the right. The path to the left is a continuation of the old familiar path the client has on. The path to the right is a new path. Take a moment to explore what it's like for the client to be standing at this crossroads. What feelings are already present? Make note!

Step 2: Experience the Expected Negative Outcomes

Invite the client to move forward along the path to the left – the old familiar way - to discover what it's like to continue in this way. As the client moves along this path, offer suggestions to remind him of the reasons he wants to make this change. This is a form of aversion therapy. For example, if the client wants to quit smoking, the path will be littered with cigarette packages, ashtrays, cigarette butts, etc. It will smell awful. It will be a dark and dreary place, a miserable place of bondage to the 'evils' of the tobacco industry. An empty, hopeless, dark, and dreary place. Build the imagery!

Don't try to make this stuff up. Any suggestions you deliver must come from the client. You're giving the client an opportunity to experience his imagined "worst case scenario." Let him show you what his expectations are by asking, "What does life look like a few months down the road?" Then you can simply reflect back to your client what he's telling you. Remember, there's nothing more powerful than the words and phrases the client is saying to himself!

Amplify the pain points. What does life look like, a year down the road, if nothing changes? Two years? Five years? What does this path eventually lead to? How does it make him feel? When the client is feeling terrible, give the suggestion, "But none of this has happened, yet." Then bring the client back to the crossroads and invite him to explore the other option.

Step 3: Experience the Positive Opportunity

The path to the right is a new path. As you guide the client down this path, give suggestions that contrast the dark and dreary path the client has just visited. Here's where you can get creative.

Incorporate images of nature like green grass, trees, and flowers. Involve all the senses. Let the client smell the fresh air and feel the aliveness of this place. It's a brighter, happier path to be on, isn't it? What does life look like a few months down this road? What about a year from now? What's changed? How much better does he feel for having made this change? What else has changed for the better? Build a sense of excitement!

Step 4: Offer The Choice
When the client is feeling really pumped with a sense of possibility, because of having explored this newer, better path, return to the crossroads. Do a quick review of the contrasting pathways. Then, once again, present the client with a choice. For example, "You're faced with a choice, here. You realize that don't you?" (pause)

"Knowing what you now know . . . which path do you *choose?*"

When the client chooses the "right" path, they are ready to proceed with the process of identifying and releasing the blocks to achieving their therapeutic goal – which means a newer, better life and all the rewards that come with having created it.

Wrapping Up

Preliminary techniques can also double as polishing techniques. You can use them to fill the void following an emotional release, encourage a more complete level of integration, deepen the healing, test the results between sessions and celebrate success. For example, when healing has occurred, you can offer statements of validation to encourage the client to allow more change.

Direct suggestions are always delivered at the end of each session, before emerging the client, to review and reinforce all the changes that occurred during the session. During your session wrap-up, remember to make whatever happened during the session relevant to the client's issue. For example, reinforce how much better the client *does* feel – mentally, physically, and emotionally. Then, connect each of these validated changes to the client's desired goal and benefits. That's what the client is paying for!

Remember, the client's expectation of success is dependent upon successfully entering into a state of hypnosis. Make sure your client is convinced that the hypnosis happened by making use of convincers during the first session. Using relaxation hypnosis in the client's first session will ensure that their first experience with you is a positive one.

If the client has been following your instructions, by the end of the first session they should be feeling more relaxed. You can then associate all the feelings and sensations of relaxation with the state of hypnosis.

Regression hypnotherapy sessions can elicit strong emotions. But it should never be so intense that the client can't speak. If you try to push through the client's emotional limits, you will only lose rapport with the subconscious mind. When that happens, it's game-over. Worse, you could result in re-traumatization.

Your job is to work with the subconscious mind – not bulldoze it into places it doesn't want to go. Remember, the subconscious mind's Prime Directive is safety. A client who is emotionally overwhelmed is in a stress response. Stress inhibits cognition which means that the client will not be able to respond effectively during the uncovering process.

This is one of the main benefits for using relaxation hypnosis in the first session. Relaxation is the antidote for stress. It shows the client that their mind is a safe place, that hypnosis is a safe place, and that *you* are a safe place to be with their feelings.

Step 1: Validate Feeling Better

Before emerging the client, verify that she is experiencing physical feelings of relaxation. Bringing the client's attention to how much better she feels will help to amplify the better feelings. You can then anchor any feelings of calm, comfort, relaxation, confidence, etc. to the state of hypnosis. For example, "Feel relaxed? It feels good, doesn't it? Notice how much better you feel. Calm. Comfortable. Relaxed. Peaceful. You've done exceptionally well. Realize what a wonderful gift you've given yourself."

Praise your client for how well she's done. Then, suggest that, from now on, she will find it easy to return to this state in future. For example, "From now on, you'll find it easy to return to this same beautiful state, quickly and easily. And each time you will go deeper than the time before, not because I say so, but because it's the nature of human beings to learn from experience. Hypnotherapy is a learning experience, a journey of self-discovery and self-healing."

Step 2: Validate Safety

Let the client have all the credit for achieving this better-feeling state. Remind her that hypnosis is safe and effective. Then, tie it to her ability to achieve their therapeutic goal. For example, "Hypnosis is a safe, effective, expedient way to create change from the inside out. Realize this state of utter calmness has been achieved by you, and no one else. No one can ever make you relax. I have simply delivered a few suggestions. It's by following my instructions that *you* have relaxed yourself. Feel proud! You've done well! Realize this is the power of your subconscious mind. It can make you into the kind of person you want to be. (Successful. Thinner. Confident. In control, etc.) This ability is going to make it so much easier for you to (realize your desired therapeutic goal). "

Step 3: Anchor Safety

Many hypnosis practitioners were taught to create an imaginary "safe place" for an emotionally flooded client to escape to. The problem is that this approach burns up precious session time, unnecessarily. It also tends to reinforce the client's resistance by encouraging their avoidance strategies. There is a better way. Instead of creating an imaginary "safe place" into which the client can escape from uncomfortable feelings and emotions, why not just make the chair the client's safe place?

This can be a real time-saver in a regression session because, should the "going get tough", all you need to do is bring the client's attention back to the chair. This allows you to keep the event on hold while the client collects themselves without reinforcing the client's dysfunctional avoidance strategies. Once the client has verified that she's feeling better, it only takes a moment to associate the more relaxed state with feeling safe and secure.

You can then anchor those feelings to the hypnosis chair. For example, "Whenever your attention goes to the sensations of your back/butt pressing down into the chair, it reminds you that you're safe here with me in my office, going deeper with every gentle breath you exhale."

Now you're all set. In the future, should you need to pull the client out of a distressing scene from the past, calmly give the suggestion, "The scene fades, and you tend to your breathing. (pause) Your attention now goes to the feeling of your back/butt pressing down in the chair. This reminds you that you're safe here with me, going deeper into hypnosis."

Step 4: Project Into the Future

If you have time, you can use Future Pacing to project these positive changes into the client's future to increase positive expectancy. Gather up all the better thoughts and feelings, walk them back to the client in the chair (going deeper), and give suggestions to integrate these changes physically, mentally, and emotionally.

Step 5: Set Up for Next Session

Before you emerge the client, set up for the next session by reminding her that she is in a process of personal change, and that her subconscious mind will continue to work on the issue after she leaves your office.

Remind her that she had done well, that she's learning how to work with her feelings in a way that allows her to heal/feel better, and that change is already occurring. Encourage her to feel proud! Then, suggest that, because of her good work, she is naturally going to *be more aware* of her feelings in daily life. Say, "I *want* you to be *very* aware of your feelings between sessions, so you can give me a report in your next session. This will give me the information I need for the next session."

Emerge the client, debrief, and then repeat the instructions to pay attention to feelings between sessions. You're all set up for the next session.

The lump, the bump, the ache, the pain – physical or emotional – is just how the subconscious mind makes an important need known to the conscious mind. The symptom is a signal. It's coming out of the subconscious mind and, like a compass, points to the source of the problem.

~ **The Devil's Therapy**

CHAPTER 3:
GOT A BRIDGE?

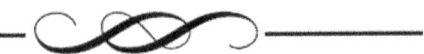

Situations in daily life can act as reminders of unresolved experiences from the past. When that happens, the person will get triggered and, either consciously or unconsciously, and relive the original event. We call that a regression. A triggering event causes the Subconscious Mind to return to the unresolved memory in an attempt to heal the problem. But the Subconscious Mind doesn't have any more resources to deal with the problem now than it did when the problem first arose. That's why it's still a problem. ~ **The Devil's Therapy**

Because the subconscious mind communicates through feelings and emotions, the first step in the healing process of regressing to the causal event is to find the feeling. All the events responsible for generating unwanted symptoms, including thoughts, feelings, and behaviors, are connected by the same feelings. When you find the feeling, you find a Bridge leading back into the event that caused it. The easiest way to find an entry-point for regression hypnotherapy is to uncover it during the pre-hypnosis interview. If you listen carefully, the client will give you everything you need to guide the process effectively.

The Steps:

1. Find it!
2. Feel it!
3. Name it!

Step 1: Find it!

To find a feeling, the client needs to feel it. Start with the body. The goal is to find an emotion. But to begin, identify physical sensations of pressure, tension, or tightness. Bring the client's attention down out of their head and into the body because that's where we feel our feelings. How does the client know they have a problem? They feel it, right?

As the client talks about the problem, watch closely for any signs of tension or tightness in the torso. When you notice it, bring the client's awareness to it. Where do they feel that feeling? Bring awareness to the physical sensations in the body. Where in the body are these sensations the strongest?

Emotions such as fear, anger and sadness are felt in targeted areas of the body, such as the throat, chest, or gut. This is what you're looking for. Focus on that feeling! "That feeling" is a subconscious signal that you can follow back to the Initial Sensitizing Event (ISE).

What's wanted?

What's missing in the client's life? What do they want that they don't have? For example: skinny body, loving relationship, confidence. Bring up the feeling that has everything to do with *not having* that by asking, "How does that make you feel?" "What emotion might that be?" 'That feeling' is a Bridge to the past.

What does the client want to get rid of? For example: fat body, fear of public speaking, habitual behavior, cancer. Bring up the feeling associated with that. How does having that problem make the client feel? What emotion? 'That feeling' has everything to do with the event that caused it. It's a Bridge to the past.

What is *not* wanted is a perceived threat that is experienced as an aversion to something specific, based on a life experience. Often, this is felt as an automatic gut-level reaction. Behind this learned response you'll find an uncomfortable emotion such as fear, anger, or sadness.

Love is a basic human need. We need it to survive. Focusing on what the client *wants* but doesn't *have* will give you access to everything that's associated with the problem. That's the Pain Package. The EFT self-acceptance phrase summarizes this beautifully by stating, "Even though I have 'this problem' (what is not wanted) ... I deeply and completely love and accept myself (want is wanted)."

What happened?

Look for a recent triggering event. What happened recently to cause the client to experience "that problem"? For example, let's say the client says, "I missed my sister's wedding reception because I was too scared to walk down the hallway!" There's the feeling!

Invite the client to tell you about that recent experience of feeling claustrophobic. Reviewing a recent event will help to bring the feeling up to conscious awareness more fully. Focusing on "that scared feeling" that has everything to do with (situation), can give you a Bridge to follow back to the event that caused it. If you want to increase the client's focus of attention, invite them to close their eyes and continue telling you the story about that recent experience.

As the client tells you the story, guide them into using present-tense language. This teaches the client how to step into an event from the past. Often, they'll regress automatically. You just need to watch for it.

Bad dreams?
When a client shares that they had a disturbing dream, treat it as you would a triggering event in waking life because, subconsciously, a dream is an actual event.

To find an entry-point for regression, invite the client to close their eyes and step back into the dream. As they share the dream narrative, facilitate the uncovering process using present-tense language, and keep the focus on the feelings being expressed through the dream. "That feeling" gives you a Bridge to the event that caused it.

Because the uncovering process encourages revivification, the client may even regress spontaneously. If it happens, yay! There's no need for a formal induction. Just step into the event and go to work!

What would need to happen?
Another way to find a Bridge to the ISE is to ask the client to describe a typical situation where the specific unwanted thoughts, feeling or behavior might arise. It could just be a hypothetical situation, such as being asked to make a presentation at work, or it could be an actual situation or event that happened recently.

What would need to happen for the client to experience that uncomfortable feeling? For example, a person with a fear of closed-in spaces might experience anxiety just thinking about stepping into an elevator. A person with a fear of heights might experience anxiety while driving over bridges. A person with social anxiety might break out into a sweat thinking about attending a family get-together.

If your client is dealing with a phobia, just thinking about being in a situation that could trigger a panic attack can be enough to bring the underlying, unresolved emotion to the surface of awareness. Watch for it because, as the client describes the hypothetical or recent event, they'll start to regress. That's the Bridge to follow. Working *with* the subconscious mind, in this way, will make regression much easier.

Provoke the Feeling

The easiest way to find a Bridge to the ISE is to provoke a feeling using non-specific language. For example, Stephen Parkhill's provocation patter is, "There's a feeling inside that you just don't like. You've tried running from it, you've tried numbing and swallowing it down (cutting it out, burning it, poisoning it, forgetting it, hiding from it, escaping it with X, etc.) *This tim*e you're going to face it. That feeling has everything to do with the problem you want to be free of. As I speak, that feeling is bubbling up to the surface. True or false, you *feel the feeling*."

Alternatively, you can use autosuggestion while stimulating the energy system of the body. For example, have the client either rub on the neuro-lymphatic release points, or tap on the Karate Chop point, while repeating a variation on Parkhill's provocation patter. "There's a feeling inside that I don't like. I've tried running from it, I've tried shoving it down, putting a lid on it, sitting on it, numbing it, swallowing it away. That feeling has everything to do with the reason I'm here. As I speak, that feeling is allowed to come up to the surface. This is *my* feeling. I'm allowed to feel it so I can heal."

You can even combine autosuggestion with Sentence Stem Completion to provoke a feeling to Bridge back on. For example, invite the client to say, "There are some things going on in my life, right now/ things that I don't like/ that are preventing me from being the person I want to be/and that makes me feel . . . (put an ending on it)." The key is to keep the client focusing on whatever is most true for them – the pain of the problem. Be creative and craft suggestions that speak directly to the needs of the client.

Find the Emotion
Physical pain often has an emotional component. Focusing on an uncomfortable sensation in the body can help you to tune into the underlying emotional signal broadcasting from the causal event. For example, focus on an area of strong tension, tightness, or pain in the body. Then, ask,

1. "Is that a comfortable feeling or an uncomfortable feeling?"
2. "How strong is that un-comfortable feeling?"
3. "If that feeling could speak, what would it say?"

Find the Thought
Fear tells us to run to safety. It's a flight-response due to a perceived threat. Ask, "What might happen?" Or offer the sentence stem, "I feel scared because (put an ending on it)." This will give you the *thought* causing that emotion.

Sadness is about loss. What or who was lost? Find the thought.

Anger is a fight response. When there's nowhere to run, anger steps in to protect. But behind anger, there's always a specific fear. Fear always comes first. When you're Bridging back on anger, the ISE will be an event that begins with a sudden, unexpected experience that triggers fear. Anger will be secondary to fear and directed toward the person(s) being held responsible for the client's pain.

Releasing the underlying fear will reduce the volume of anger. As a result, the client will feel more in control and experience greater mental clarity. If they then discover that their angry feelings were caused by a misinterpretation of the event, their anger will dissolve completely.

Anger is about protecting boundaries – our own, or someone or something we care about. It might be due to a perceived injustice, betrayal, or an assault that caused injury. Who is responsible for causing that hurt? Keep in mind that, where there is anger, there is also love. Who needs to be forgiven to find the love?

Step 2: Feel it!
During the intake process, as the client talks about herself and the problem, invite her to tell you about a recent triggering event. What happened recently to cause her to feel "that feeling?" Or what would need to happen for her to experience "that feeling?" As the client tells the story, keep your eye on what's happening in their body. Pay close attention for signs of discomfort. For example, tension in the shoulders, tightening of the fists, tears, flushing, clenching the jaw, swallowing, accelerated breath-rate, etc.

The moment you notice any signs of discomfort, bring the client's attention to it. Focusing on the feeling will help to amplify the feeling, giving you a stronger Bridge to the past. And once the client has found the feeling in the body, you'll know they're feeling it.

The next step is to isolate "that feeling" in the torso region of the body. That tense, tight feeling in the gut might be a "scared" feeling, or it might be an "angry" feeling. But you won't know what's coming up until the client tells you what they are experiencing by naming the emotion. Ask, "What emotion might that feeling in your (throat/chest/gut) be? Mad? Sad? Scared? Or something else?"

> **Watch the Body**
>
> *Some clients will show up in a state of hyper-arousal. For them, it's their habituated state. They're stuck in a chronic stress response that generates physical tension and anxiety. For example, a client presenting with anxiety, or who is apprehensive about experiencing hypnotherapy, may already be "worked up" before they show up on your doorstep.*
>
> *How can you tell? Conduct a simple test. When your client arrives for their session, take their hand. Is it warm or cold? The physical symptoms of a stress response include cold hands, excessive perspiring, dry mouth, heart pounding, shallow breath, knot in the stomach, queasy stomach, tension headache, loss of appetite. These are the body's natural response to a perceived threat. If the client's hands are cold on a warm summer day, you'll know they're in a stress-response.*

What just happened?

Anytime a client shows signs of discomfort during a process, pause what you're doing to find out, (a) what emotion the client is experiencing and (b) what just happened to trigger that feeling. For example, during the preliminary intake the client may begin to cry. Clearly, the client is experiencing an emotion. When that happens, pause, right there, and bring the client's attention to "that feeling."

What was the client just talking about? What just happened? What's the story? How did that make the client feel? What emotion? Where do they feel that in the body? How strong is that feeling? "That feeling" is a Bridge to the past. You know what to do!

Abreaction?

An abreaction is not an irrational reaction – it's an emotional regression. Something just happened that acted as a reminder of an unresolved event from the past. This re-stimulated the old, familiar feeling that the client doesn't like. When this happens, the client is already regressing. Use it!

What happens when you squeeze a grapefruit? What's on the inside comes out, right? The same thing is true of emotions. During your sessions, pay close attention to the client's responses because even the most seemingly grownup client can get triggered. And when a client gets triggered, they'll abreact. The feeling that the client is experiencing might be very uncomfortable, overwhelming, even, but it's not new to them. They've felt that feeling before and *they don't like it*! You didn't cause it. It's not what's happening in the present moment that's the problem. The client brought that feeling in *with* them and it has everything to do with their presenting issue. Ask, "Is that feeling (in your gut) new or familiar?" The client will tell you they've had that feeling before. There's the feeling! *Name* the emotion. Then follow it back!

Step 3: Name it!

When a person lets themselves feel the feeling in the body, and then names the authentic emotion associated with that feeling, it starts to lose its power over them. The problem is that emotionally illiterate clients tend to use words like "stressed," "upset," "anxious," or "depressed."

While saying, "I feel upset" is a socially acceptable way to get some distance from the actual feeling, "upset" is not an emotion. It's a thought. Similarly, "inadequate," "stupid," "foolish," "not-good-enough," "inept," "defeated," "trapped," and "hopeless" are not emotions. When a client uses a thought to describe a feeling, recognize this as their learned strategy for avoiding uncomfortable feelings. While this can provide the client with a much-needed sense of safety and control, you won't get very far if you try to Bridge back on a thought like "anxiety" or "stressed." Teach your clients to recognize, experience and name actual emotions like fear, anger, and sadness because a real emotion is a signal coming out of the event that caused it.

To locate the ISE, you need to find the feeling in the body and then name the specific *emotion*. Encourage your clients to use words like "scared," "afraid," "angry," "mad," and "sad." "That scared feeling in the gut", or "that angry feeling in the throat" or "that sad feeling in the heart" has everything to do with a specific unmet need that was experienced during a specific event, at a specific age. "Terrified," "frightened," "pissed," "rage," and "heart-broken" are all acceptable because they describe authentic emotions being experienced in the body. Naming the specific emotion will help the client reclaim their right to *have* feelings while giving you a more targeted Bridge.

If the client has difficulty naming the emotion, ask, "If that feeling could speak, what would it say?" This should provide you with clues as to the actual emotion you're dealing with. For example, fear arises when we're facing a threat. It's there to let us know that we need to take action to protect ourselves. Sadness is a feeling that recognizes a loss. Anger points to an injustice or betrayal, or the need to avoid getting hurt by protecting our boundaries.

Remember, emotions are never the problem. Avoiding emotions is the problem. Keeping a lid on our feelings only makes the problem worse by creating internal pressure. We call that pressure "stress." Guide the client to name the emotion before you begin Bridging back. "That feeling" is what's calling for healing. Once the ISE has been located, the purpose for having that uncomfortable emotion can be identified and resolved for good.

How strong is "that feeling?"

You need a strong Bridge to regress back on. When the client is clearly feeling an emotion, invite them to locate it in the body. For example, "Where do you feel 'that feeling' in your body?"

Once you have located it in the body, *quantify* the feeling by asking, "On a scale of 1- 10, where 10 is the worst that it has ever been, how *strong* is that feeling?" (You need a 7 or higher to Bridge back on.) If it's less than a 7, ask the client's permission to bring that feeling up to at least a ten. Then, use an amplifying count to increase the intensity of emotion. Amplifying the feeling will give you a stronger Bridge and, therefore, a clearer path to the causal event.

Troubleshooting the Bridge

Not sure if they're feeling it?

Some clients are not very emotionally expressive. If you're not sure if the client is experiencing the feeling, ask, "True or false, you feel the feeling?" Verify that the client is following your instructions before proceeding. If the client responds, "true", quantify the feeling. How strong is it? Then, guide the client to name the emotion.

If the client responds, "false", back up a step. Find the feeling that has everything to do with the client's presenting problem. You can use provocation patter or ask, "What would need to happen for you to experience that uncomfortable feeling?" Once you find the feeling, quantify it. If necessary, amplify the feeling. Make sure you have a strong Bridge to follow back to the causal event.

Can't find a feeling?

Children naturally feel their feelings. The only people who feel nothing are dead! *Not*-feeling, or not being able to name an emotion, is often the result of conditioning early in life. As a result, some of your clients may be disconnected from their emotional life. This is a common pattern with people who are suffering from depression.

You can help to restore their natural ability to feel their feelings by teaching the client how to find, feel and name an emotion.

1. Locate the feeling in the body. Where in the body is that feeling strongest? (Throat, chest, gut?)
2. Focus on *that* feeling.
3. Name the emotion. (Sad, mad, scared, or something else?)
4. Quantify the feeling. On a scale of 10, how strong is it?
    a. Less than 7 = amplify.
    b. More than 7 = Bridge back.

Client won't allow the feeling?

If the client is experiencing an emotion but is resistant to allowing more of the feeling to come up, focus on making it safe for uncomfortable emotions to come to conscious awareness. You can use Muscle Response Testing (MRT) or ideomotor signaling to identify the specific objection(s). Alternately, you can use Stems Completion

Exercise and autosuggestion to deliver set up phrases which help to identify and remove psychological reversals[11].

1. Even though I don't deserve (to get over this problem) ...
2. Even though it's not safe ...
3. Even though it's just not possible ...
4. Even though it won't benefit me ...
5. Even though I'll be deprived ...
6. Even though I'm not willing to give myself permission to change anything ...
7. Even though I'm not willing to do what's necessary to (address the issue)
8. Even though I don't want to change ...
9. Even though I don't want to (get over this problem) ...

The key is to customize your suggestions to the specific needs of the client. For example: "Even though **it's not safe** to feel this feeling ... I choose to let it come up strong within me ... *because* what I can feel I can heal ... so I accept this feeling."

"Even though **it's not safe** to feel this feeling ... I let myself go where I need to go ... see what I need to see ... hear what I need to hear ... feel what I need to feel ... *so I can heal* ... because I deeply and completely accept myself ... And all my feelings."

"Even though **it's not safe** to feel this feeling ... I can feel it ... I'm allowed to feel it ... And I'm allowed to release it ... because I deeply and completely accept myself."

In some cases, you may want to grind down further to access the specific objection. You can do this easily by repeating the setup phrase

---

[11] Psychological reversal is an EFT term for any resistance to change. According to Gary Craig, when a psychological reversal is present, it literally blocks progress.

and adding "because." For example, "Even though I don't want to (get rid of the problem) because . . ." might take you back to "it's not safe" or "I'll be deprived".

In some cases, a secondary gain issue could be brought to light. For example, "I don't want to get over this problem because I'll be abandoned by the people who care for me." To grind down, add the next Stem, "The thought 'I'll be abandoned' makes me feel . . ." What emotion? Focus on "that feeling." The feeling will provide a Bridge to the event that caused it.

Remember, you need a strong Affect for Regression to Cause. If there's an objection to allowing the feeling, there's no Bridge to the ISE. In this case, focus on releasing the block.

CHAPTER 4: WHY HYPNOSIS?

In a therapeutic setting, hypnosis is really the least important part of the session. People don't pay for hypnosis - they pay for results. You don't want to waste a lot of your session time on the induction. You want to get the client into hypnosis and then get to work on the problem. Before you do this, you need a client who is convinced that the hypnosis happened and who can enter a state of somnambulism very quickly. ~ **The Devil's Therapy**

The Elman Induction is a works-in-the-drawer induction[12] that can be adapted to almost any client. The Elman is my induction of choice because it's a very step-by-step approach, it has all the tests and convincers built right into it, and it only takes a few minutes to get a client into somnambulism. Plus, you can easily convert it into a relaxation type induction, a rapid induction or even an instant induction.

The key is to adapt your approach to the needs of each client. If what you're doing isn't working, try something else. Really, the only way you can fail is by giving up.

---

[12] In other words, everything is built into the induction process.

The Steps:

The Elman induction follows the following five-step process.

1. Eye Closure
2. Eye Lock Test
3. Fractionation
4. Hand Drop Test
5. Numbers Challenge

Troubleshooting Eye Closure

The first goal in the Elman Induction is eye closure. This may seem like no-big-deal. Just tell the client to close their eyes, right? Wrong. The client thinks they're paying for *hypnosis*. This means that they need to be convinced that they've been hypnotized. If you don't satisfy this need, doubt can set in and block you. Doubt shows up as resistance. You may not even realize what all the fuss is about but, when doubt sets in, you'll find yourself in a wrestling match with the client's conscious mind. Why not get rid of the doubt by satisfying the client's expectation to be hypnotized? Then, you can focus on what the client is really paying you for, which is the results. The way to do this is to formalize your induction.

Formalize the Induction

The induction process is really a ritual. Formalizing your induction means giving it a clear beginning and a clear end. This lets the client know when the hypnosis is starting and when it's over. The Elman Induction begins with eye closure. Rather than allowing the client to just close their eyes, make it a ritual with clearly defined steps. It's not about getting the eyes to close. It's about establishing an agreement-frame. This gives you a way to test to make sure that the client is going to follow your instructions.

You also need to give your hypnosis session a clear ending by using a formal count-up to emerge the client from hypnosis. Don't just say, "Whenever you're ready, you can open your eyes." That's too wishy-washy. Take charge of your session right from the start and do away with doubt by giving your induction a clear beginning and clear ending.

Between the closing of the eyes and the emerging from hypnosis, you can then use the built-in tests and convincers in the Elman Induction to provide proof that hypnosis really happened.

The following five suggestions will put you in charge of the healing process right from the start.

1. Look at my hand.
2. Take a nice deep breath in, really fill up your lungs.
3. Hold it, hold it, hold it ….
4. Now, as you exhale relax and close your eyes.
5. And let the body begin to relax.

Watch the client's response to each suggestion. If the client accepts the first suggestion, they're more likely to accept the next suggestion.

Step 1: "Look at my hand."
Every suggestion serves a purpose. The first suggestion tells the client to do something specific. "Look at my hand."

If the client looks at your hand, you can see that they're following your instructions. What you're doing is teaching the client to pay attention to the things you tell them to pay attention to. Throughout the process of regression hypnotherapy, you'll be asking the client to notice things that they don't normally pay attention to – like uncomfortable feelings. This is setting up for that to happen.

Step 2: "Take a deep breath in."
The next suggestion is, "Take a nice deep breath in, really fill up your lungs." When the client takes a deep breath, you can see that they're following your instructions. Filling up the lungs serves a purpose. It creates a little physical tension in the body. On the inbreath, the shoulders will lift a little. The chest will expand a little.

Step 3: "Hold it, hold it, hold it . . ."
When the client holds their breath, you'll see the body tense up a little. Holding the breath for a few moments increases the tension, making the client more aware of the physical sensations of tension in the body. That's useful.

Step 4: "Now, as you exhale, relax and close your eyes."
As they release the breath and close the eyes, the body will release that little bit of tension created by holding the breath.

Step 5: And let the body begin to relax.
Relaxation is not hypnosis. The client is not in hypnosis, yet. But the suggestion to allow the body to relax brings the client's attention to the feelings and sensations of physical relaxation coming on. That's what you want. The releasing of the breath will automatically be accompanied by a feeling of relief.

The body will naturally start to relax because the client has let go of the tension they were holding onto. As a result, the suggestion to "let the body begin to relax" will be completely congruent with what the client is already experiencing. This builds trust because what you're saying is true. It's also a non-verbal suggestion that letting go is how the client will feel better. This is a suggestion you're going to reinforce when it comes time to do the emotional release work.

Repeating the suggestion to let the body relax, throughout the deepening process, can help the client to release a lot of pent-up stress. As a result, the session is more likely to end with the client feeling noticeably better than when they first began. This can help to build confidence in the healing process by providing evidence that change is possible – if you use it.

Many clients are unaware of just how much physical tension they've been holding onto. If the client experiences a deeply relaxing first session, before emerging them, bring their attention to how much better they feel. Deliver a few suggestions to reinforce the fact that change is already occurring. This isn't just something you're saying! They *know* this is true because they can feel it!

To build positive mental expectancy toward the desired results, suggest that these changes will continue as you continue to work together. Then offer a few suggestions to remind them of all the benefits for having created change.

Not following instructions?

If the client is not following instructions, guess who's taking charge of your session? The client's conscious mind. Don't let that happen! The moment the client fails to follow instructions, stop right there, address whatever is happening, and then start over. For example, I've had clients close their eyes before I gave the instruction to do so. If the client closes their eyes before you give the instruction to do so, say, "Wait! Don't start without me!" Right away, they'll open their eyes and look at you in surprise.

Don't make a big deal of it. Treat it lightly but make them start over. This may seem like a trivial thing. Usually, it's because they've experienced hypnosis before and think they know what to expect. Nuh-uh! This is going to be different! But here's the main problem - you haven't even started the session and, already, the client is taking control. They're not following your instructions. They're hi-jacking the session. Don't let that happen. Take charge of the process and teach your clients how to behave in their sessions with you, right from the start. It will make your job so much easier!

Anxiety client?

High-anxiety clients can be challenging. They're not being difficult. It's just that their brain is firing on twelve cylinders. This means that you need to work quicky to stay ahead of it.

If the client is so wound up that they can't keep their eyes closed, a relaxation induction isn't going to be effective. Either switch to a rapid induction or use tapping to calm down their energy system. Tapping is a natural induction process that has a lovely calming effect, and you can use it to release some of the internal tension. When that happens, the client will begin to drift into a natural state of hypnosis, and you can switch to a more formal induction procedure.

Troubleshooting the Eye Lock Test

The eye lock test is not a test for hypnosis. It's a test for compliance. Some people think that compliance means "control", but all it really means is "cooperation". If the client is willing to cooperate by following your instructions, you have permission to guide them into hypnosis. You need that.

The problem with the eye lock test is that it's a test the client can fail. If you give the instruction to "check to make sure the eyelids won't work", and then the eyes open and the client looks at you, you've got a problem! Worse, the client may be giving themselves a suggestion, "It's not working." Sometimes the problem is that you weren't clear enough with the instructions. Sometimes the client wasn't paying attention. Sometimes the client is flat-out challenging you by thinking, "Make me!" That's resistance!

Whatever the reason might be, now you have to deal with it, and that can take time. If you don't deal with it, you're going to have more problems to deal with later. Fortunately, this can easily be avoided by troubleshooting the problem.

Does the client understand?
Make sure the client understands what you're asking them to do. What you're asking them to do is relax the eyelids to the point they won't work. The critical suggestion is, "When *you're sure* that they won't work, test to *make sure* they won't work." You're not asking them to try to open their eyes. You're asking them to (a) relax the eyelids so much that they just won't work, (b) make sure that they're that relaxed, that they just won't work, (c) check to make sure that they won't work. That's it. Repeat these instructions, then ask the client, "Do you understand?"

Do you have the client's attention?
Make sure the client is paying attention. Hypnosis requires the client to focus attention on your instructions. It's not something that *you* do. It's by paying attention and following your instructions that *they* will achieve a beautiful state of hypnosis. Make sure the client understands that you can't do it for them.

The only thing that will prevent a person from entering a state of hypnosis is conscious mental activity. Hypnosis requires setting aside thinking, analyzing, and trying to figure things out. Make sure the client is paying attention to your instructions because the moment they start thinking, "This isn't working …" it's game over. They're back up in their head, which means that they're not paying attention to your instructions. They're following their own mental chatter.

Are your instructions reasonable?

If the client has *failed* to follow your instructions, that's okay. It's early in the induction process. Often, all that is needed to establish compliance is to make following your instructions reasonable. Remember, the induction process requires the conscious mind to relax. The client accomplishes this by setting aside conscious mental activity. The problem is that the conscious mind needs a reason for everything. You can satisfy this important need by making your suggestion reasonable, then gaining permission to repeat the process.

> **Remember:** *Your best overall strategy is to prevent problems from happening, in the first place. Never move on to the next step until the client successfully completes the step you are on. When you do bump into a problem, stop right there! Resolving it becomes the next logical step in the client's healing process. In this way, you can walk the client right out of the problem.*

First, let the client know that (a) hypnosis is a skill that can be learned, (b) they are *learning* how to take themselves into a state of hypnosis (c) so that they can enjoy all the benefits. Second, give the suggestion, "Human beings learn through trial and error. So, let's do that, again." Then start over from eye closure. When you get to the eye lock test, make the desired response reasonable by suggesting, "When you relax a muscle, it can't do anything. So, if you have followed my instructions to relax the eyelids, they won't work. They'll just remain relaxed and remain closed."

Who is responsible for the results?
Nothing is going to happen without the client's permission. If the client isn't willing to follow your instructions, you're both going to be frustrated. You must-must-must make the client responsible for the results. For example, when you give the instructions to relax the eyelids to the point they won't work, tell the client to (a) "double the relaxation there," (b) "keep doubling the relaxation in the eyelids until *you're convinced* that they're that relaxed, that they just won't work," (c) "Keep doubling the relaxation until *you're sure* they won't work."

Never conduct a test that your client can fail. The eye-lock test is easy to make fail-safe simply by adding the suggestion, "I can't do this for you. If those eyelids were to open, it would simply mean that you need to double the relaxation a few more times. Keep doubling the relaxation until *you're sure* they won't work. When you feel that those eyelids are that relaxed, that they just won't work, *take a nice, deep relaxing breath in* and, as you release the breath, go deeper." Now, all you have to do is watch for the inbreath. When the client takes a deep breath and exhales, give instructions to go ahead and conduct the test. Nice, right?

Subtle response?
If you're working in low-light conditions, you may not be able to see a subtle response to the test such as a slight flutter of the eyelids. You need to see the response so that you can immediately deliver the command, "Stop testing and go deeper relaxed." The simplest solution is to instruct the client to raise their eyebrows when they conduct the

test. For example, "In a moment, I'm going to ask you to check to make sure that they're so relaxed that they just won't work. And if you have followed my instructions, you'll find that the *eyebrows go up and down*, but the eyelids remain relaxed, and remain closed."

When the client conducts the test, all you have to do is watch for the eyebrows to raise, and you will be able to easily observe the response to your suggestion. Try this out for yourself. Close your eyes. Relax the eyelids to the point they won't work. Then, conduct the eye-lock test while raising the eyebrows. See? Fail-safe!

Troubleshooting Eye Fractionation

In the traditional Elman Induction, once the client has passed the eye lock test, the next step is to fractionate. Eye fractionation is the process of opening and then closing the eyes to create the illusion of emerging and re-entering hypnosis. Fractionating can be used as both an induction and deepening technique. The more times you repeat it, the more deeply the client will go into hypnosis.

Following eye closure and passing of the eye lock test, the suggestion is given, "In a moment, we're going to do that again. Only, *this time*, you'll be able to go ten times deeper relaxed." The client is then instructed to open the eyes, then close the eye, and go ten times deeper, anchoring the sensations of relaxation to deepening into hypnosis.

Here's the problem. The client has just successfully *relaxed* the eyelids to the point that they won't work. Opening the eyes necessitates removing the relaxation from the eyelids. Why not just compound the relaxation that's already been established in the eyelids?

Instead of instructing the client to open their eyes, simply engage their imagination. Have them bring their awareness back to the eyelids and relax them ten times deeper relaxed. Then, conduct the test, again. You can then instruct the client to send *this* quality of relaxation throughout the body to establish a deeper level of physical relaxation. (Later, you can use the deepening sensations of *physical* relaxation as evidence of hypnosis happening.)

Troubleshooting the Hand Drop Test

If the client is following your instructions, they should be experiencing sensations of deepening relaxation. But how do you know if they're following instructions?

The hand drop test is a covert test which allows you to check to make sure the client is relaxing. It's a covert test because the client doesn't know it's a test. You're secretly testing their response to suggestions. For example, "In a moment, I'm going to lift your hand and drop it. I'm only going to lift it a couple of inches but *if you have followed my instructions*, this arm will feel heavy to me like a piece of marble or stone, but loose and limp like a wet dishrag."

When you conduct the test for the hand drop, lift the arm by gently grasping the client's wrist with two fingers. You only need to lift the arm up a few inches, but the arm should feel heavy when you pick it up.

Next, give the wrist a little wiggle to check for flaccidity. The wrist should be droopy and wobbly. If it's rubbery, the client is following instructions. This is the desired response – heavy, loose, and limp like a rag doll. Reward the client with a few words of praise. For example, "That's good!" Or "You're doing great!"

Next, lift the arm a little higher to test the elbow. Again, the arm should feel heavy and rubbery. Once again, reward the client with a few words of praise before moving onto the shoulder. Test the shoulder by lifting the arm up and down a few times. The shoulder should follow the arm. Loving touch is very comforting and the body will naturally respond to it by relaxing.

If you have permission to touch, place your hand gently on the client's shoulder and press down gently. The shoulder should feel slightly soft and spongy when you press down. You can then offer a suggestion to encourage the shoulder to relax a little *more*.

Floaty?

When you lift the wrist or arm, it should feel heavy. If the client's arm seems to float up by itself, the client is not following instructions. They're helping. The client is anticipating your lifting the arm up. They need to stop doing that. Firmly instruct the client to stop helping. For example, "Don't help! Let me do all the lifting!"

Teach the client to follow your instructions by delivering step-by-step instructions. For example, give the instruction to "relax the wrist, let it go loose and limp." Then, test. When the client relaxes the wrist, offer words of praise, and move to the next step. Give the instruction to "relax the elbow, heavy, loose and limp." Test that the elbow is relaxed. Then, repeat with the shoulder. Whatever the client gives you, use it.

If the client is following your instructions, you'll feel the arm will get heavier and the wrist, elbow and shoulder will take on a more rubber-like quality.

If the client is still trying to help, switch to arm catalepsy[13]. When it comes time to do the hand-drop, simply give the suggestion to relax the stiffened arm, and the arm-drop will happen naturally.

Rigidity?
If the wrist is rigid or stiff, give the suggestion to relax the wrist. For example, "Let it go loose and limp." The client may be following instructions, but some clients need to be taught *how* to relax.

A client with arthritis or bursitis may not be able to relax the wrist or shoulder. If the client has had a shoulder injury, they may unconsciously be holding onto tension as a protective measure. In this case, the shoulder will feel stiff or rigid but the wrist will be relaxed. Remember, you're testing to make sure the client is responding to your suggestions. Any evidence of relaxation is a pass for the client. Praise their success!

Watch it!
You can drop the hand onto the arm of the chair or into the client's lap. But when you drop the hand, let it drop only a few inches and it will act as a deepener. Even though the client knows it's going to happen, it generates a small shock which tends to deepen the client's state.

Be especially careful when working with male clients. If you drop their hand into their crotch, they will emerge themselves! Make sure it drops onto their leg or the arm of the chair. A more maternal approach is to wiggle their hand a little, then place it gently onto their leg. As an added deepener, press down gently as you give the suggestion in a lulling tone to *relax e-v-e-n more* . . .

---

[13] If you're working online, you can use arm catalepsy for the hand-drop.

If what's happening is perceived as safe, the brain will generate the all-clear. If there's a perceived threat, it will sound the alarm. This signal takes the form of stress hormones like cortisol, adrenalin, and norepinephrine. These hormones put the body on red alert. They also don't feel good because the body is responding to a threat. Stress hormones tell the body to get ready to take action and ensure your survival either by fighting or fleeing. That's the subconscious mind's Prime Directive – survival.

~ **Radical Healing**: *Hypnosis Practitioner's Guide to Harnessing the Healing Power of the Educational Pre-Talk*

CHAPTER 5: GOT A REAL REGRESSION?

You need somnambulism to revivify an event. Regression is not merely thinking about or remembering a past event. It is a reliving of the experience – seeing, hearing, sensing, and feeling – just as it was the first time. The client steps into the event, and it's all happening now. This allows the underlying cause of the client's symptoms to be brought to conscious awareness. ~
The Devil's Therapy

Real regression requires somnambulism. This is because somnambulism facilitates revivification[14] of past events, not merely recall. This is why you need to test for state. The test that is built into the Elman Induction is the Numbers Challenge, also known as the Losing the Numbers Test. This is a test for the threshold of somnambulism. To maintain the state, once you have induced it, you must then deepen the client below the threshold of somnambulism.

The Steps:

1. Count down slowly from 100.
2. Say the number out loud, then relax it out of the mind.

---

[14] Revivification means "to relive".

3. Exhale and relax the mind and body together.
4. As the mind relaxes, all the numbers relax out of mind.
5. After just a few counts, all the rest dissolve and disappear.
6. When they're gone, say, "All gone."

The Numbers Challenge is conducted by suggesting to the client to begin counting down slowly from 100. They're instructed to say the number out loud, then relax it out of their mind so that after a few numbers, they will have relaxed all the numbers out of their mind. When they're all gone, the client is to let you know. For example, "In a moment, I'm going to ask you to begin relaxing the mind, in the same beautiful way you have relaxed the body. Here's how you'll do it. You'll begin counting down from 100. You'll say the number out loud. Then, as you exhale, relax even more. And as the body relaxes, the mind relaxes. As the mind relaxes, it only takes a few counts, so that by the time you reach 97 or 96 . . . maybe sooner, you will have relaxed all the rest of the numbers relax right out of your mind. It feels so good. And when they're gone, just let me know by saying, "All gone.""

The keys to successfully facilitating the Numbers challenge are:

1. Repeat the instructions. Make sure the client understands what you want them to do.
2. Demonstrate how to count down slowly, starting with 100. Pace your count to the client's outbreath.
3. Once you have delivered the instructions, avoid using the word "number" to ensure you do not reinstall the numbers.
4. Be patient. Give the client time to lose the numbers. The client's attention needs to be on relaxing the numbers out of the mind. This can take a little time.

Troubleshooting the Numbers Challenge

Client is hurrying?
If the client seems to be rushing through the numbers in a race to get to the finish line, you need to slow them down. Speak softly and slowly as you instruct the client to (1) Say the number very s-l-o-w-l-y, then (2) take a deep, relaxing breath in and, (3) as you exhale, take a moment to relax the mind, allowing "all the rest" to dissolve and fade away to nothing-nothing-nothing. (4) And notice how good that feels.

To slow things down, even further, you can use autosuggestion by instructing the client to add the words, "deeper relaxed" after each count. For example, "100 . . . deeper relaxed . . . 99 . . . deeper relaxed, etc."

Alternately, have the client count backwards in threes. For example, "100 . . . 97 . . . 94 . . . 91." This will increase the client's conscious attention on finding and then releasing the number, thereby deepening the hypnosis.

You can also insert intermittent patter into the process by talking quietly in the background. This overloads the conscious mind by giving it too many things to pay attention to. For example, "As you continue to go deeper, with every gentle breath that you exhale, I'm going to be talking in the background. You'll be aware of everything. But I want to you to focus on relaxing, and as the body relaxes, the mind relaxes, so that you can begin to enjoy that wonderful *mental* relaxation, that feels so good."

Client: "Ninety-four . . ."

CH: (softly) "That's right . . . And as you exhale, now, you'll find it easy to relax them right out of your mind. You're aware of everything, and yet you are not aware. Listening with your subconscious mind, while your conscious mind is drifting farther and farther away, not listening. Your conscious mind is drifting farther and farther away, and not listening. You're doing great."

Client: "Ninety-three . . ."

CH: (soft, lilting tone) "Gooood. Your subconscious mind is very aware, and listening, and hearing everything while your conscious mind is becoming more and more relaxed, very relaxed, and peaceful. You're allowed to relax peacefully, more comfortably, now, because your subconscious mind is taking charge, and when this happens, it feels so good, they just fade away to nothing-nothing-nothing, allowing your subconscious mind to do all the listening."

Client: "Ninety-two . . ."

CH: "Your subconscious mind knows, that's right, and because your subconscious mind knows, your conscious mind does not need to know and can drift, more comfortable, now, deeper relaxed, as all the rest fade to nothing-nothing-nothing."

Client: "Ninety-one . . ."

CH: "Just like little boats sailing off into the horizon . . . or clouds drifting far, far away . . . Dissolving into nothing, nothing, nothing. You can just let them all go, now, it feels so good . . ."

Client: "Ninety . . ."

CH: "That's right. Dissolving away, dim and distant, it doesn't matter if you forget, your subconscious mind remembers everything that you need to know. And you can let your subconscious mind listen and remember while your conscious mind drifts, drifts, far-far-away. That's right. Just push them out, now. You don't need them. And when they're all gone, you can nod or say yes."

(Continue with your patter until the client indicates "yes.")

All gone? (Client confirms.) That's good. And as you continue to listen to me, with your subconscious mind, your conscious mind can rest peacefully and sleep, sleep, sleep, deeper and deeper r-e-l-a-x-e-d.

High Achiever type?
If your client is a goal-focused, achiever-type, they may try to go for the gold by counting all the way down to zero. In this case, instead of having them count backwards from 100, have them start counting *up* from one. As there are infinite numbers, this presents an unachievable goal which they'll soon give up on.

Instruct the client to go *more deeply relaxed* with each number they say. The suggestion of "more" is congruent with the increasing count and, because there are unlimited numbers in front of them, the client's tendency to strive for the finish-line is effectively defeated.

If you want to slow them down a little, have them take a deep breath after each number or say the words, "Deeper relaxed." Then, suggest, "With every gentle breath that you exhale, go-more-deeply-relaxed."

Client stops counting?
If the client stops counting, quietly ask, "All gone?" If the client nods, move to the next step.

If the client does not respond, ask if they are having difficulty speaking. Aphasia can be a symptom of profound depth. In this case, you can have the client nod, use ideomotor signals, or simply instruct the client to come back up to a level of hypnosis where they can speak.

If there's still no response, test to see if the client has fallen asleep. It happens. If the client is sleep-deprived, their subconscious mind may grab the opportunity to relax beyond the hypnosis into natural sleep. Give instructions to open their eyes on the count of three. If the eyes don't open, gently rouse the client and switch to a rapid induction.

Client starts snoring?

If the client starts snoring, don't assume that they have fallen asleep. Snoring can be a result of physical relaxation. Without changing your tone or rhythm, say, "In a moment, I'm going to ask you to open and then close the eyes. If that's okay with you, nod your head."

If the client nods, they're in hypnosis. Instruct them to open their eyes, then close the eyes. Then, give the suggestion to stop snoring.

If the client doesn't nod their head, wake them up, then use a rapid induction to reinduce hypnosis.

Not entering hypnosis?

All hypnosis is self-hypnosis. If the client is not entering into hypnosis, there's a reason. You need to find out what that reason is. Have the client open their eyes and have a chat.

What's happening? Are there some fears or misconceptions about the process that the client hasn't disclosed?

Does the client understand that hypnosis is achieved by following your instructions?

Does the client understand that hypnosis requires setting aside thinking, analyzing, and trying to figure things out?

Has the client ever been hypnotized before? If so, by whom? What happened? If the client is experiencing apprehension or anxiety regarding the process, it may be due to a previous experience they haven't told you about.

If the client is over the age of 65, ask if they have ever been hypnotized before. For example, by a dentist, doctor, psychologist, psychiatrist, etc. This is rare, not to mention unethical, but there may be a hypnotic seal in place. You can bypass it by letting the client hypnotize herself. (Remember, all hypnosis is self-hypnosis.)

First, have the client close her eyes and think back to the time she went into hypnosis at the dentist. Then, invite her to bring you into the scene by telling the story using present-tense language.

Begin with arriving at the (dental) office. Day time or night time? Inside or outside? Alone or with someone? Help the client to associate into the scene by using all their senses.

Next, move to the moment when the hypnotist begins to do the induction. As the client describes everything as it is happening, she will return to a hypnotic state. You can then remove the seal by giving the suggestion, "Whenever you want to enter hypnosis with me, or anyone you trust, you can do so quickly and easily. And each time, you will go deeper than the time before."

Analytical or anxious type?

Relaxation hypnosis is not appropriate for every client. Relaxation inductions give the client too much time to think. As soon as they start thinking, "Is it happening?" you've lost the battle. Their conscious mind has been activated and will effectively prevent the client from entering a state of hypnosis.

If your client is highly analytical or anxious, relaxation hypnosis may be too slow. The solution is to switch to a rapid induction. Work quickly to stay ahead of that brilliant mind of theirs.

The following induction can get a client into verifiable, deep somnambulism in less than a minute. It's perfect for analytical types because it overloads the conscious, thinking mind[15].

To set up, instruct the client to stare at a spot above eye level. This generates eye fatigue. Then, give the instruction that when you say "NOW" the client will simultaneously do the following four actions.

"One, concentrate on your right hand and imagine that it's getting heavier, like a sopping-wet dish rag or a piece of marble or stone.

"Two, begin lifting your left hand in the air as slowly as humanly possible - less than a millimeter per second. (There are 20 mm to an inch.)

"Three, notice that the eyes are getting heavier and heavier.

"Four, when those eyes are that heavy, that you just can't keep them open any longer, let them close down, and begin counting backward, out loud, starting with 100. Count slowly and softly, and with each

---

[15] Overload Induction by Cris Johnson, author, speaker, entertainer.

number, relax more and more mentally until after just a few numbers, all the rest just disappear. When they're all gone, just nod your head and go deeper."

Repeat the instructions. Then, give the command, "NOW" and remain silent. Let the client do the work. When the client's eyes close, it will take less than a minute for them to nod their head, signaling to you that the rest of the numbers are gone. Remember to deepen immediately.

A More Reliable Test

While the Numbers Challenge is built into the Elman Induction as a test for the threshold of somnambulism, it's not necessarily a reliable test for state. Just because the client tells you that they have lost all the numbers doesn't mean they're gone. Some clients will try to please you by telling you what they think you want to hear. As a result, the Number Challenge makes a better test for compliance than for depth of state. A more reliable way to induce and test for somnambulism is to use eye fractionation followed by a covert test.

Because eye fractionation mimics the experience of emerging and reinducing hypnosis, you can get a person into deep hypnosis very quickly. As a result, eye fractionation can shorten the time it takes to guide a person into somnambulism. But you still need to test for state. The following covert test for somnambulism[16] gives you a much more reliable test for somnambulism. It does require some skill to get the timing down, but it's so reliable that I swapped it out for the Numbers Challenge, entirely.

---

[16] Gerald Kein, Omni-Hypnosis Training

The Steps:

Step 1: Setup
This process begins after establishing eye closure, conducting the eye-lock test, and the test for physical relaxation. Then, give the instruction, "In a moment, I'm going to count from one to three. On the count of three, let those eyes open. I'll say the word, "Sleep!" and snap my fingers like this (snap!). The moment you hear the snap, **and not before**, close your eyes and double the relaxation."

Repeat the instructions. Make sure the client understands.

Step 2: Three Count
"Let's begin. 1, 2, 3 ... (Wait for eyes to open.) Sleep! (Snap fingers!) . . . and go deeper."

Step 3: Conduct Test for Compliance
Immediately deepen by gently placing your hand on the client's forehead and rolling the head gently from side to side. "As I gently rock your head just allow yourself to go loose, limp and relaxed."

If the muscles in the neck are relaxed, you'll be able to randomly guide the head movement. This is another test for compliance.[17]

Step 4: Repeat Three Count
"Once again, I'm going to count to three. On the count of three, those eyes will open. *When you hear the snap* (snap fingers), instantly, automatically, spontaneously those *eyes close down*, and you go even deeper. 1, 2, 3 ... (Wait for eyes to open) Sleep! (Snap!) ... And go deeper."

---

[17] If you're working online, you'll have to forgo this covert test.

Step 5: Repeat Head Roll Deepener

"Let yourself melt down even deeper now. Drifting down deeper with each and every breath you exhale. Every word takes you deeper. Every thought takes you deeper. Every sensation. Deeper and deeper. You'll find that every time I do that you will go deeper and deeper into hypnosis. So, let's do that again.

"1, 2, 3. Sleep!" (Snap!) ... and go deeper."

Keep repeating until the response becomes automatic or the client is struggling to get the eyes open. The trick is to establish a lulling rhythm. For example, "1, 2, 3, Sleep! (Snap!) and go deeper. Beautiful. And again. 1, 2, 3, Sleep! (Snap!) and go deeper."

Step 6: Test for State

Once the client is responding to your suggestions on cue, you can conduct the eye fractionation test by inserting a pause between the two and the three-count. For example, "1, 2, (pause)... 3, Sleep! (Snap!) ... and go deeper."

There should be *no anticipation* of the count of three. The response should be automatic. If the client is not anticipating the three-count, the eyes will remain closed until you say, "three." This indicates that the client is now entering into a state of somnambulism. When that happens, give the suggestion, "Every part of you is responding beautifully, now. Perfectly now, as you are learning how to allow that Part of you that makes all changes to respond effortlessly to *all* my suggestions. And you'll find that, as I continue to talk to you, all these suggestions are working at a very deep, deep level. And all changes will occur automatically, *not because I say so* but because this is what you desire now."

Deepen Immediately

Once the client passes the test for the threshold of somnambulism, deepen immediately. You need to deepen below the threshold because the client's state will naturally lighten during the session. Examples of effective deepening techniques include:

- Deepening Count, doubling or tripling the relaxation
- Counting with or without intermittent suggestions
- Period of Silence
- Pacing the client's breathing with or without shoulder press
- Hand-drop or shoulder press
- Sounds utilization
- Pyramiding inductions

Pyramiding Inductions

You can stack one induction on top of another. This is called "pyramiding" the induction. Once you have induced a light state of hypnosis, a subsequent induction will act as a deepening technique. Pyramiding your induction can get you uber-deep hypnosis. (Eye Fractionating is an induction technique. When stacked on top of the Elman Induction, it acts as a deepening technique.)

Sounds Utilization

Once you have deepened the client into somnambulism, you can utilize potential distractions as deepeners. For example, "From this point on, every gentle breath that you exhale can take you deeper. Sounds around you will not bother or disturb you. The only sound that interests you is the sound of my voice. Every word guides you deeper, and deeper relaxed. Any sounds that do arise will only help and guide you to go deeper. For example, the sound of the traffic passing by on the street . . . or the sound of a phone ringing in another room . . . realizing these are the ordinary everyday sounds of this environment. You'll be aware of those things but the only thing that interests you is the sound of my voice. And as your attention returns to the sound of *my* voice, you will go deeper into hypnosis."

Want a built-in deepening technique during regression? Use the sound of the client's voice as a deepener. For example, add, "Even the sound of your *own* voice can take you deeper."

Regression hypnotherapy is a journey of self-discovery and self-healing. During a regression session, there's a lot going on behind the scenes that you know nothing about. The mind processes information a lot faster than a person can speak. As a result, everything that's happening in a regression session isn't necessarily going to be shared with you. Clients can withhold information that might be relevant to their healing because they don't think it's important or are too embarrassed to tell you about it. They may not feel comfortable sharing it with you right away.

~**Ditch the Script**: *Get Everything You Need from the Client for Successful Hypnotherapy and Set Up to Wrap Up with Results*

CHAPTER 6: GOT A STRONG BRIDGE?

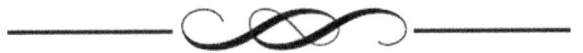

The way to access a strong Bridge is to hone in on it. You need the conscious mind to be focused on one thing. Keep the focus on just one thought, or one feeling, or one specific sensation in the body. Remember, that thought or feeling or sensation is a signal that is coming out of the event that caused it. It acts like GPS. All you need to do is keep the conscious mind focused on that, and it's like targeting the ISE. – **The Devil's Therapy**

Every problem is the result of a life experience. The experience responsible for the client's presenting issue – physical, mental or emotional - is called the Initial Sensitizing Event (ISE). This is the experience that "sensitized" the client to be vulnerable to specific triggers. The ISE is merely the beginning of a story that has been developing over time. That story has to do with a specific pattern of perceptions, thoughts, and feelings. Subsequent events which, in any way, presented as a match to the pattern trapped in the ISE, served to re-stimulate and reinforce the underlying problem. This is why symptoms tend to get worse over time. The goal of regression hypnotherapy is to locate and release the problem in the ISE. Bridging back powerfully is how we get there.

The Steps:

1. Find a Bridge.
2. Validate the feeling.
3. Quantify the feeling.
4. Amplify the feeling.
5. Test for the feeling.
6. Focus on "that feeling".

Step 1: Find a Bridge

While you can use a Cognitive Bridge (thought) or Somatic Bridge (physical sensation) to regress to the ISE, Affect Bridge (emotion) is the preferred method for age regression. This is because every event is linked emotionally. Emotion is the language of the subconscious mind and, as such, gives you a clear signal leading right back to the event that caused it.

You can shorten the path to the ISE by using a directed regression to begin with. Then, switch to Affect Bridge. For example, during the pre-hypnosis interview, identify the earliest event the client can consciously recall in which they experienced the problem. Guide them back into that consciously remembered event and have the client replay the event while in hypnosis. Conduct the preliminary uncovering procedure to help the client associate into the event, then bring up the emotion. Once the client has found and named the emotion, you can use it to Bridge back to the ISE. This gives you a shorter path to the ISE. Much quicker.

If you don't have a consciously remembered event, that's okay. You can launch from the here-and-now by using a non-directed approach. For example, to bring up a feeling to Bridge back on, use the following patter with gusto! "There's a feeling inside that you *just don't like*. That feeling has everything to do with the reason you're here. As I speak, that feeling is coming up to the surface. *Let that happen.* This is the perfect place for that. You've tried running from it, you've tried stuffing it down, putting a lid on it, numbing, and swallowing it away. *This time* you're going to face it. As I speak, that feeling is allowed to come up powerfully within you."

Test to make sure the client is responding to your suggestions by testing. "True or false, you feel the feeling." If the client's answer is "true", immediately ask, "Where do you feel that feeling in your body?" (Proceed to quantify the feeling) If the client's answer is "false", what happened? The purpose of this patter is to provoke an uncomfortable feeling. To do that requires an authoritarian, energetic tone. You need to stir the pot. Are you using a soft, lulling tone?

If your tonality is congruent with the intention to evoke an uncomfortable emotion, it could be that the client is not *allowing* the feeling to come to the surface of awareness. When you bump into a block, that's resistance. You just need to find out what the specific objection is and address it. Back up a step to your educational pre-talk and establish the contract. Remember, the contract (a) requires the client to allow uncomfortable feelings and memories to be a part of the process, and (b) allows you to hold the client accountable for the result.

Remember: *Never proceed to the next step until the client has successfully completed the step that you're currently on. When you bump into resistance, that's where the work begins. If you try to make the client fit your protocol, you'll get nowhere. Adapt your protocol to the client and you'll succeed. Nothing builds success like success. Teach your client how to be successful working with you.*

If the client is bumping into fear, that's okay. Remind the client that "that feeling" has everything to do with the problem. Allowing the feeling to come to awareness gives you a path to the cause of the problem. Reassure the client that you've got this! If necessary, use autosuggestion, with or without tapping, to release the fear of facing the feeling. For example, "Even though it's not safe to feel this feeling . . . I'm allowed to feel it . . . this is my feeling . . . I choose to let it come up strong within me . . . because I deeply and completely accept myself . . . **If I can feel it, I can heal it**[18] . . . This time I *let* myself feel it . . . so I can heal."

Step 2: Validate the feeling.

Once the client indicates that she is feeling the feeling, validate it, then locate the feeling in the body. For example, "There's the feeling! That feeling has everything to do with the reason you're here! Where do you feel that in your body?"

Client: "In my tummy!"

CH: "There's the feeling! That feeling in your tummy . . . is that a comfortable feeling or an uncomfortable feeling?"

Client: "Uncomfortable! It hurts!"

CH: "Ooooh! It hurts! That feeling is allowed to be there! It has everything to do with (presenting problem). What emotion might that feeling in your tummy be? Sad, glad, mad, scared or something else?"

Client: "Scared! I feel scared!"

---

[18] This is an incredibly powerful suggestion borrowed from the title of a book by Dr. John Gray.

Step 3: Quantify the feeling.
You need a strong signal to follow back to the event that caused it. If you try to follow a weak Bridge back, you'll end up having problems you just don't need. Either the client will bail out, they'll lose the feeling, or they'll revert to thinking and remembering.

To ensure that your Bridge doesn't fizzle out, ask the client to *quantify* it by taking a Subjective Unit of Discomfort (SUD) on "that (scared) feeling in your (gut)." For example, "On a scale of one to ten, where ten is the worst that feeling has ever been, how *strong* is that feeling?"

Step 4: Amplify the feeling.
You need at least a seven to regress back on. If the client says, "It's a twelve, you're good to go. If the SUD level is less than seven, you're best to amplify the feeling. But to do that, you need the client's permission. For example, "We need that feeling to be *at least* a ten. Would you be willing to let it come up to a ten so that we can heal it?"

With the client's permission, you can now use an amplifying count. For example, "Focus on that feeling in your (gut). As I count from one to five, let that feeling come up powerfully within you, understanding that "that feeling" is allowed to be there. Your permission to allow that feeling to be felt and released is what allows you to heal. Understand?"

"One, there's the feeling. It's that feeling inside that you just don't like. You can feel it in your body. It doesn't feel good.

"Two, coming up powerfully within you, now. You *feel the feeling* bubbling up to the surface.

"Three, coming up more powerfully, now. You *feel the feeling*, like a dam bursting forth . . .

"Four, and on the next count, *there's the feeling*, as strong as you've ever known it before, and

"Five! There's the feeling. Say, "I feel" and put an ending on it!"

Where attention goes, energy flows. While you are counting upward, watch the client's responses to your suggestions. If you observe physical changes, mention them during your count. Feeding your observations back to the client will help to amplify the feeling. For example, "There's the feeling! I can see that you're feeling it! Your breathing is getting stronger. Your face is getting red. You feel the feeling! Three, coming up more powerfully, now, etc."

Step 5: Test for the feeling.
At the count of five, test to find out what emotion you're going to Bridge back on. This takes all the guesswork out of the process.

CH: "Five! There's the feeling. Say, "I feel" and put an ending on it!"

Client: "I feel scared!"

You now know that (a) the client is immersed in the feeling and (b) you're Bridging back on the feeling of fear. If the client says, "I feel sad", the Bridge you're following is the feeling of sadness.

Once you have brought a feeling to awareness, located it in the body, identified what emotion is expressing, and quantified the strength of the feeling, you have a solid signal leading back to the ISE. All that's left to do is give the instruction to stay focused on "that feeling."

Step 6: Focus on "that feeling".
The goal is to locate the ISE because that's the first time the client ever experienced "that feeling." But there may be multiple emotions

involved in a client's issue. **You can only follow one at a time**. This is the key to effective Bridging. Focus on one thing at a time. Don't change horses, mid-stream. Follow "that feeling" all the way back to the event that caused it. Resolve it completely at the ISE.

If the client bumps into another emotion while you're Bridging back, reassure them that you'll take care of it, "in a minute." Make a note of it but bring their awareness back to the Bridge you're following. For example, if you were following fear back, keep the focus on "that scared feeling in your tummy". If you were following sadness, keep the focus on "that sad feeling".

The one exception to this rule is anger. If you Bridge back on anger and it changes to fear, follow the fear. All negative emotion is rooted in fear. Anger is a secondary emotion. It comes after the fear. Fear is the initial response to a perceived threat. When there is no escape route, anger will step in to protect. Resolving the initial fear will reduce the anger trapped inside, making it much easier for the client to release. This will make the forgiveness phase much easier.

Lily Pad Approach

The ISE is the weakest link in a chain of events which, together, are responsible for causing unwanted symptoms. Often, the ISE turns out to be no big deal because events in childhood involve responses and decisions which lack the benefit of emotional and cognitive maturity. This can make resolving the problem at the ISE much easier on the client – and you – but because the signal coming out of the ISE is weaker than that of subsequent events, the subconscious mind is more likely take you to an SSE. This is because later events generally have more emotional intensity which is generating internal pressure which the subconscious desperately wants relief from.

If you give the instruction to go back to the "first time," don't assume that the subconscious is going to follow your instructions. You are most likely going to be disappointed with your results. Sometimes, it's just a Bridge too far to get back to the ISE in a single leap. Sometimes, there's an SSE that has so much pressure trapped inside it that the subconscious mind wants relief – NOW! In any case, you'll have much better control over the regression process if you use the following Lily Pad approach. In addition, this approach will provide you with a list of SSEs through which you can later grow the Child up.

Bridging Patter

Whether you're Bridging back from the here-and-now, or from a consciously remembered event, keep the client focused on the feeling in the body. Then, use a rapid count down to "an earlier event". This is a much easier task for the subconscious mind to accomplish because it's only a short hop from the present moment to an earlier event. For example, "There's the feeling! I'm going to count from five down to one. On the count of one, your mind has you in an *earlier* scene, situation, or event that has everything to do with "that feeling."

"Five, going back in time.

"Four, to a scene, situation, or event of significance to "that feeling."

"Three, arms and legs may be growing smaller, now, as your mind takes you further and further back.

"Two, moving right into that event of significance. The scene grows vivid, real, and clear. And on the next count, there you are, as real as the first time.

"And ONE. There you are. Say, "Here I am (wait for client to repeat). And I feel (put an ending on it.)""

The first bounce back may take you to an SSE that occurred a few years ago, or you may bounce back to an event in childhood. Much of this depends on where you're starting from.

If you're Bridging back on the emotion the adult awareness of the client is experiencing, there will be more events between the ISE and the here-and-now.

If you're starting your Bridge in an event earlier on the client's timeline, such as a consciously remembered situation in childhood, the length of the Bridge will be shorter, and there will be fewer SSEs to traverse.

If there's an SSE with a big emotional charge to it, there's a good chance it will snag the subconscious mind during the count-back. As the objective is to do all the work in the ISE, there's no need to spend a great deal of time on an SSE. All that's required is to maintain rapport with the subconscious mind.

The Steps:

1. Bridge to an earlier time.
2. Conduct preliminary uncovering.
3. Test for ISE
4. Promise to come back and take care of the problem.
5. Continue bridging back to the ISE.

Once you land in an event, conduct a little preliminary uncovering to find out what happened, and validate the feeling. Then, conduct the test for the ISE. Reassure the subconscious mind that you're going to take care of this. Then, continue Bridging back until you find the ISE. In this way, you can hop from one lily pad to the next until you achieve the ISE.

> **TIP:** *In the first session, if you have educated the client about childhood events during the pre-talk, then guided the client through the hypermnesia exercise, you could find yourself within easy reach of the ISE. You're already in childhood, which gives you a much shorter Bridge to follow. If you're lucky, you could locate the ISE very quickly. Nice right?*

Troubleshooting the Bridging Process

Client Won't Regress?

Regression happens naturally, given the right conditions. The only thing that can prevent it from happening is conscious mind interference. Is the client in hypnosis? Conscious mental activity will prevent a person from entering into hypnosis, blocking access to the part of the mind that is responsible for memories and emotions.

Have you conducted a test for depth? Depth isn't a constant. Unless the client is immersed in a strong emotion, the tendency will be for the state to lighten. Remember, once you have tested for the threshold of somnambulism, you need to deepen immediately before attempting to Bridge back to an earlier time. Then, keep the focus of attention on the feeling.

Did you bring up the feeling powerfully? Remember, you need a strong Bridge for regression. Weak emotion – weak Bridge. No emotion – no Bridge.

Is the client taking medication? If they use alcohol or marijuana to help them relax or get to sleep this may be an issue. For example, marijuana can block the client's ability to enter a state of hypnosis or produce short-term results. Some clients are taking prescription medications.

For example, anti-depressants are designed to block a person's ability to feel. This is not usually a block to regression, but it does mean that you need to override the dampening effects these drugs have on emotions. Work quickly, deliver suggestions with authority, and make sure you have a strong Bridge by amplifying the feeling. Then, take a SUD. Make sure it's coming up powerfully before you proceed with the count-back.

Lost the Bridge?

If the client brings up the feeling and then loses it, your Bridge has fizzled out. In this case, you need to start over. The question is – why did it happen?

Is your patter clear and direct? If your suggestions were unclear the client won't understand what they're supposed to do. This can bring in the conscious mind to protect. Clear direction provides safety.

Is your delivery brisk and authoritative? If your regression patter is too slow the client will lose focus. They could even fall asleep. Remember, regression doesn't require relaxation. It requires somnambulism. While relaxation can be useful in the first session, when it comes to Regression to Cause, focusing on relaxing the client can be counterproductive. Use a more dynamic approach. Provoke the feeling, amplify as needed, keep the client's attention on "that feeling" and Bridge back with gusto. Work quickly and authoritatively. Remember, you need a strong Bridge to get to the ISE.

Have you established a contract for regression? The contract should give you permission to "go there". Without it, nothing is going to happen. You're asking the client to let you guide them into uncharted territory and to face uncomfortable feelings. The Contract promises safety.

Is the client thinking? The most common problem is conscious mind interference. Either the client is consciously trying to remember or trying to figure things out. Analysis-paralysis will block the regression. Say, "True or false, you feel the feeling." (This is delivered as a statement, not a question.)

If the client responds, "False", start over. Remind the client that the only thing you're interested in is the feeling. That feeling is an emotion. It's a signal coming out of the event that caused it. Establish a Contract. Establish somnambulism. Bring up a strong emotion and Bridge back with authority.

If the client responds, "True", focus on the feeling. Quantify the feeling. Amplify as needed. Bridge back with authority.

Lost the feeling on the Bridge?
If you find a feeling, Bridge back to an earlier event, and begin the uncovering process only to have the client report, "Nothing," don't panic. Respond matter-of-factly with, "Sometimes 'nothing' is something. Focus on that 'nothing' feeling." Then, ask "Where in the body is that 'nothing' feeling expressing?"

If "that nothing feeling" is located in the gut, the chest, or the throat, you're on target. Validate it by saying, "There's the feeling!" Instruct the client to focus on "that feeling." How strong is that "nothing feeling." Having the client describe to you how they are experiencing "that feeling" will amplify awareness of the feeling.

How young does the client feel as they're feeling that (descriptors) feeling? Sometimes, the problem is simply that the Child doesn't have a word for an uncomfortable feeling. For example, "nothing" could be a feeling of emptiness or aloneness.

As the client focuses on that "empty feeling", they may realize that what they're feeling is actually sadness, or hurt, or scared, or something else.

Client Doesn't Want to "Go There"?
Nobody wants to go there. Remember, you're dealing with learned defenses which serve the purpose of safety. That's why the client needs you! But if you try to push the client some place they don't want to go, it puts you into a wrestling match with the client's subconscious mind. When that happens, *you* become a threat.

You need cooperation, not obedience. Back up a step. What does the client need to feel safe in proceeding?

If the client is feeling apprehensive about what might be revealed in an event, this could be subconscious interference. It could also be an indication that you are on the threshold of identifying the underlying cause of the client's issue! Recognize that a block is the "way through." You're knocking on a door behind which answers can be found. You just need to find a way to get the door open. This is where the work is -- resolving the resistance to facing and feeling painful events from the past.

Option 1: Have a chat with the subconscious mind and use your best lawyering skills to convince the subconscious to grant permission for the client to "go there." For example, "I don't know if this has anything to do with why you're here. I *do* know that it came up. *This* is the way through. *This* is where your miracle lies! You have the choice to *follow my instructions*. Listen, if your conscious mind could have thought your way through, it would have! You're smart! You're intelligent! And you're here! You can continue to live the life you're living. You already know where your life will be . . . one year, five years from now . . . doing what you've been doing. Or . . . you can *follow my instructions*."[19]

Option 2: Come in through the back door by using a positive regression. Instead of requiring the client to face a "forbidden feeling", instruct them to go back to a time *before* they ever knew what it was like to feel bad, sad, mad, scared, etc. Uncover and amplify the positive feelings and emotions in that earlier scene to facilitate ego-strengthening. Then, you have a choice of how to proceed from there.

a) You could simply ask the Child if "that problem" the client came to see you about has been experienced, yet. You could then move forward or backwards to locate the ISE.

b) You could gather up the positive thoughts and emotional energies in the earlier event and bring them back to just *before* the event that presented a block. You can then install these positive energies into the Child before moving forward into the event.

c) You could Bridge back to the first day of life, bring in Adult Consciousness to welcome the Child into the world and prepare them for "the trouble" that lies ahead on their timeline. You can then instruct the subconscious mind to send the positive changes forward through the client's timeline up to present time. This will give you a more resourceful client to work with while weakening SSEs.

---

[19] Stephen Parkhill patter

Whopper SSE?

While finding the roots of the problem in childhood can help you to get quicker results, the client must have sufficient clarity with which to make sense of what happened in the ISE. Time spent clearing an SSE can give you a client who is better-equipped to face a traumatic childhood memory, and who is better able to connect the dots to the presenting symptoms. This will get you better results.

If you bump into a deep pocket of pain in an SSE, deal with it. Just don't make the mistake of trying to suggest away the feelings so that you can continue onto the ISE. That will only cost you rapport with the subconscious mind. It could even make things worse. Recognize that the client's subconscious mind is showing you an event of significance because it trusts you to provide some much-needed relief. Honor that. This is an opportunity to clear a path to the ISE by releasing the pressure in the SSE.

You don't have to completely clear an SSE. Just release enough of the internal pressure to allow you to uncover what happened to cause the client so much distress. The subconscious mind naturally generalizes all learning. As a result, clearing some of the emotional charge trapped in a significant SSE can generate important insights which can then be used to transform the ISE.

Once you have reduced some of the pressure, reassure the client's subconscious mind that you will come back and take care of the problem - *in a minute*. Then, gain permission to continue Bridging back to the ISE. Clearing the ISE will reduce the energy flowing into subsequent events, making these later pockets of pain much easier to deal with. As a result, when you come back to the (Whopper) SSE, it will be significantly easier to resolve.

Make sure you keep your promise to return to the event. There may be other aspects trapped in that event that are calling for resolution.

Troubleshooting Tips

Regression hypnotherapy is a very step-by-step process. Before applying a therapeutic technique, think about what needs to happen next.

If you try to push beyond the client's readiness, it puts you at odds with their subconscious mind.

Before you begin a therapeutic process, have a clearly defined goal in mind. If you don't know where you're going how can you know how to get there?

The question to hold top-of-mind is -- what's the next logical step? This will help you decide which tool or technique to use. Should you deepen further? Should you provoke a feeling? Should you amplify that feeling? Should you release it or regress into it? The answer is - it depends.

It depends on the client. It depends on what their therapeutic goal is and how ready they are to proceed to the next step.

CHAPTER 7: GOT THE REAL PROBLEM?

T*he subconscious mind is the conscious mind of the past. What this means is that when you regress a client into an event in childhood, you are speaking to the conscious mind of the client at that age.* ~ **The Devil's Therapy**

In any given moment, the conscious mind is being bombarded by information that's coming in from the environment. The problem is that the conscious mind is limited. It can only process about forty bits of information per second. The subconscious mind, on the other hand, can process about 20,000,000 bits of information per second. That's 500,000 times more powerful than the conscious mind[20].

It isn't that the information isn't getting in. It's that very little of it is being processed consciously. As a result, the Adult/conscious mind doesn't have the whole story. The purpose of the uncovering procedure is to bring to consciousness the story behind the client's presenting issue.

---

[20] https://spdrdng.com/posts/conscious-vs-subconscious-processing

The uncovering procedure focuses primarily on what happened in the Initial Sensitizing Event (ISE) because that's the experience that generated the symptom-requiring pattern. To identify this pattern entails identifying the age at which this event occurred, the cast of characters (Players) involved, the specific feelings and emotions still trapped in the event and the decision(s) that were made, based on the perceptions of the client at that time. Often, this event involved some kind of trauma in childhood.

Common childhood traumatic experiences include:

- Abandonment:
- Abortion/Miscarriage
- Abuse (Physical, Sexual, Emotional, Verbal)
- Accident
- Alcoholism/Addiction
- Anxiety/Panic
- Birth Trauma
- Death
- Divorce
- Domestic Violence

The Key Elements

Like a story, every event has a beginning, middle, and an end. The beginning of the story is whatever was happening *before* the actual traumatic experience occurred. This means that, if you have successfully located the ISE, if you go *before* the event, the Child will be feeling good, okay, safe, happy, peaceful. Then, something will happen to change that. That's when the drama begins to play out.

This is where you can uncover all the key elements that are responsible for causing the client's unwanted symptoms. The problem is not what happened in the event. The problem has to do with the stress-response. Young children are easily overwhelmed by feelings and emotions. They also lack the maturity with which to make sense of the world of people and things around them. The real problem has to do with how the Child interpreted what was happening. As a result, the Child felt overwhelmed. This resulted in a disruption to the energy system of the body.

There is always a critical moment in the event where the emotional energy comes to a peak. This moment is what the client would describe as "the worst part." Think of this energy peak as the turning point in the story. Everything has been building up this moment. It's like the crest of the hill. If you release the emotional intensity before and after this energetic crescendo, the nervous system will start to relax and reset. When this happens, the client will have more clarity regarding what's happening. As a result, uncovering the details will become easier.

- What's happening?
- Where is it happening?
- Who is involved?
- What sensations are being triggered in the body?
- What do those things make the Child think?
- What emotions are surfacing?
- What does the Child need or want (that wasn't available at that time)?

The reason the ISE is still a problem is because the subconscious mind doesn't realize that the event is over. This leaves the Child trapped in the emotional energy of the event, still trying to find a solution. This is the fundamental problem - the subconscious mind only has the resources of the Child. But decisions made at this time can form beliefs about what to expect - from self, others, and life in general - because of this experience.

Aspects that can be calling for resolution include:

- Things said . . .
- Things done . . .
- Things seen or heard . . .
- Thoughts that arose in response to those things . . .
- Feelings associated with those things . . .
- Impressions of self or others . . .

How does the event/story end? Once you have uncovered the key information, ask the Child, "Looking ahead in life, what does life look like because of those things that just happened?"

The Steps:

1. Set up for the uncovering process.
2. Step into the event.
3. Name the emotion(s).
4. Uncover the age.
5. Uncover the unmet need(s).
6. Identify the cast of characters.
7. Test for ISE.
8. Identify trapped feelings.
9. Identify decisions.
10. Uncover the layers.

Step 1: Set up for the uncovering process.

Your regression sessions will unfold much quicker if you set up for the uncovering procedure before you guide the client into hypnosis. Use the following pre-hypnosis exercise to teach your client how to respond to uncovering questions during a regression session.

CH: "Before we begin, let's do a little exercise to show you how to respond during the session. Okay?"

Client: "Okay."

CH: "Whenever I ask you a question, I want you to *answer quickly, without thought*. Understand?"

Client: (nods)

CH: "Just let that thinking part of you stay off to the side, somewhere, and let yourself *feel the answer*. That's what we want. There's no right or wrong answer. Just give me your *first impression*. Whatever comes up first, okay?"

Client: (nods)

CH: "Okay. Let's just do a little practice to make sure that you understand. This will only take a minute. Go ahead and close your eyes, and let yourself go inside, and just *notice how it feels*. (pause) Now, *first impression* (pause), does it *feel* like its day time or night time?"

Client: "Day time."

CH: "Good job! First impression, does it *feel* like you are inside . . . or outside? *First sense…*"

Client: "Inside."

CH: "You're doing fine. First impression, does it *feel* like you're alone ... or with someone?"

Client: "With someone."

> If the client says, "alone," they are most likely identifying a feeling of aloneness. The fact is that the client is not alone; they are with you. But just stay with the exercise, for now.

CH: "Beautiful. Open your eyes. (Make eye contact.[21]) That's all there is to it. Whenever I ask you a question all you need to do is (a) focus on how it feels and (b) answer quickly by giving me your first impression. Understand?"

If the client responds with an incorrect answer - for example, the client responds "nighttime" when it's mid-day, or "outside" when they're inside your office - it may be that their mind has associated back to an event from the past. When this happens, continue to validate the client's response. This will demonstrate to the client that there are no right or wrong answers, only thinking or feeling responses. Remember, the purpose of this exercise is to teach the client to (a) answer without thinking and, (b) stay focused on the feeling.

Consciously the client knows that it's daytime, that they're inside, and that they're with you. But their subconscious mind knows why they're seeing you. It's possible that the client has regressed into a scene from

---

[21] Want to employ the 'hypnotic gaze'? Focus on the area between the client's eyebrows. To the client, it will seem like you are making eye contact and you'll be able to maintain your gaze without being distracted by their responses.

the past. That's okay. Just complete the exercise, then conduct a little debriefing process to explore what just happened. For example, "A moment ago, your mind had you somewhere. What came up?"

As the client describes the scene or memory that came to mind, you can then decide how best to use it. For example, you can use it to illustrate how the subconscious mind naturally associates to earlier events. This is a natural ability that you will use as you work together.

If the scene or memory has an emotional quality to it, you could use it to teach the client how to release a feeling to feel better.

If the associated feeling is strong, you could begin the regression work right there. Simply have the client close their eyes and step back into the scene. Repeat the uncovering procedure to bring up the feeling for Affect Bridge and you'll be "off to the rodeo"!

Step 2: Step into the Event

Bridge back to "an earlier time." Then, teach the client how to step into the event and revivify it before Bridging back further. This helps to deepen the hypnosis while you conduct a little preliminary uncovering work and create a map[22] of the series of SSEs leading back to the ISE.

To help the client step into an event, give the instruction during your count-back, "And on the next count, here you are, as real as the first time. You see what you see, you hear what you hear, you know what you know, and you feel what you feel. And ONE. *Be there.*" Then, instruct the client to repeat after you, "Here I am. And I feel (put an

---

[22] See Session Mapping in The Devil's Therapy.

ending on it.)" This is a test that allows you to make sure the client is still connected to the Bridge.

As soon as the client steps into the feeling in the event, proceed with the uncovering work. For example, the client says, "Here I am... and I feel scared!" Give the suggestion, "Stay focused on "that scared feeling. First impression, does it feel like it's daytime or nighttime?" Continue with the uncovering process to identify the key elements. Then, conduct the standard test for the ISE.

Sometimes, the client will know, immediately, where their Mind has taken them. When this happens, you can encourage revivification of a memory by teaching the client to use present tense language. This will help to paint the picture of the scene/situation. Once the client steps into the event, more of the details will be made clear. For example, "3, 2, 1. Be there! First impression, does it *feel* like its daytime or nighttime?"

Client: (hesitant) "...Daytime?"

CH: "Good! Does it *feel* like you're inside or outside?"

Client: "... Inside?"

CH: "Good! Does it *feel* like you're alone or with someone?"

Client: "... Feels like I'm alone..."

CH: "How *young* might you be that you're feeling alone?"

Note: "How old are you?" can be interpreted as interrogative and is incongruent with the Bridging suggestion to go to a younger age.

Client: "Really little!"

CH: "Good job! How young might you be that you're really little?"

Repeating the client's own words helps to increase revivification.

Client: "Just a baby!"

CH: "First impression, how *young* do you feel? Days, weeks, months …?"

Client: "Weeks?"

CH: "Good. There's a Part of you that knows how young you are. First impression, how many weeks?"

Client: "Six?"

CH: "Say, 'Here I am / six weeks old / and I feel alone …'"

Note: Another effective way to increase revivification is to use Autosuggestion. Having the client repeat the impression helps them to take ownership of their perceptions. This will usually bring clarity about what's happening.

Client: "Here I am / six weeks old / and I feel alone."

CH: "I feel alone because (put an ending on it.)"

Adding the word "because" will give you more details about what's causing the Child to feel uncomfortable.

Client: "The family is in the other room."

CH: "That's right. What do you want that you feel so alone?"

Perhaps, the most important question you can ever ask the Child is, "What do you want?" Children are seldom asked what they want or need. Needs that go unmet cause pain.

If, at any point during the uncovering process, the client bumps into a block to awareness, you can gently tease out the next important piece of information by stacking the client's responses into a mini-review question. For example, "What's happening that you're here in the kitchen with Mom feeling scared?"

Step 3: Name the emotion(s)
"The two Rs in R2CH are regress and release. *Regression* gives access to information trapped in the causal event. *Releasing* removes the subconscious requirement for symptoms. The secret to achieving a lasting result lies in the releasing.[23]"

Naming the actual emotion the client is experiencing will help you to get a more complete release of a feeling. But to name the emotion, you need to consider what is age-appropriate for the client. The younger the Child, the more limited and simpler their emotional vocabulary will be. A toddler's emotional expression will be limited to basic emotions. For example, sad, mad, hurt, scared, alone. As the Child grows and matures, so, too, does their emotional vocabulary.

Step 4: Uncover the age.
What is the age of the client in the Event? How young might the client be in the event? The ISE is almost always before the formation of Critical Faculty of the Mind which occurs around the age of five. Prior

---

[23] The Devil's Therapy: Hypnosis Practitioner's Essential Guide to Effective Regression Hypnotherapy

to this, the mind of the Child is wide-open to verbal and non-verbal suggestions, and experiences are downloaded into memory without the benefit of critical thinking. These memories are not recordings of truth or fact. They simply represent how the Child interpreted what was happening, based on the knowledge and maturity of the client at the age at which the event occurred.

If the client uses words like "small," "little," "powerless," "weak," or "helpless," you are very likely addressing a young Child.

If the Child is not sure, or cannot give you their age, ask, "First sense. Does it feel like you're standing, sitting, or lying down?"

If they're lying down, you may be dealing with an infant. In this case, ask the client to describe what they might be lying on. This will help the client to build the scene piece by piece, allowing the facts regarding the event to be revealed.

If the client reports that they are standing or sitting, gently tap the back of their hand and say, "Show me. How many fingers?" Young children often do not know their age but they can show you how many fingers they are.

If the Child is an infant, ask, "First sense. How young might you be - days, months, or years?" Once you have identified this, you can zero in on the specific age incrementally. For example, if the client reports that they "months old", ask, "How many months?"

If the client reports a feeling of floating or says, "tight," this may indicate that she has regressed to the womb. Ask, "Is it light or dark?" Then ask, "Does it feel like there's a lot of room around you or a little?" Then, "Does it feel like you are alone or with someone?"

If the answer is "with someone," find out who the Child is with. (First sense!) If it's Mom, ask the Child to *feel* the answer to the next question, "Are you inside or outside Mom?"

If the client spontaneously realizes that they're inside the womb, often this will come as a surprise. This sudden realization will usually bring the scene to clarity making the uncovering process much easier.

Step 5: Uncover the unmet needs(s).

What are the unmet needs of the Child? The cause of the problem has to do with an unmet need. What was missing that the Child wanted or needed? The most fundamental problem is that the Child had to cope with the experience on her own. What was needed was support. With no one there to help her make sense of what was happening, the Child felt isolated, vulnerable, and overwhelmed. Bringing in the client's adult consciousness, to accept and support the Child *before* anything "bad: happens, can help to resolve this fundamental problem.

Children are dependent upon others to meet their needs. For some reason, the person the Child depended upon to provide safety and security was absent. Who was the Child's primary caregiver? Usually, this is Mom. Whoever the Child wanted in their moment of distress, that person will need to be forgiven. In fact, anyone who comes to mind during the ISE needs to be forgiven. For example, the Child witnessing Dad having an affair feels bad because this would be hurtful for Mom.

Step 6: Identify the cast of characters.

Who are the Players? Who might the Child be with? The things that were said and done by Players in the event made impressions on the Child. These impressions generated thoughts and feelings which are contributing to the client's symptoms. As a result, these are the people the client most needs to forgive to be set free from their influence.

- Who is there?
- What is their relationship to the client?
- What role are they playing in the event?

Even peripheral players are important. If the client mentions someone while telling the story, this indicates that this person has been associated with the story and may need to be forgiven, as well.

Step 7: Test for the ISE.
Have you landed in an ISE or SSE? The goal is to get to the ISE - the "first time" the client ever felt "that feeling". For example, "that" fear, or "that" sadness, or "that" anger. Emotions are very specific.

While ISE theory suggests that the ISE is before the age of five, the ISE is often to be found before the veil of amnesia forms around age three. There can be exceptions, of course. Any traumatic event can act as an ISE at any age. But regardless of the age at which the traumatic event occurs, the feeling will be new. It will come as a surprise. For example, "Where did that come from?" as opposed to, "Uh-oh ... Not again!"

The standard ISE test is the Feeling Test, "That feeling in your (gut) . . . is that a new feeling, like a surprise? Or an old familiar feeling like, 'oh-boy, here we go, again'?" Even when the client reports that the feeling is "new," give the instruction to "go back to the first time you felt that feeling." Most of the time, the subconscious mind will show you an earlier event.

The question, "new or familiar?" is not the test for the ISE. The test is the client's response. If the client goes to an earlier event, you know you landed in an SSE. Repeat the preliminary uncovering procedure, conduct the test, again, and keep Bridging back unto you locate the ISE.

If the client bounces back to the same event, it's safe to assume you have located the ISE and can proceed to uncover the details about what happened in that event.

Another test you can use to verify the ISE is the Safety Test. ISE Theory states that *prior* to the ISE the Child will feel good, safe, and secure. Therefore, if you go just before the story starts to play out, and the Child is feeling okay, you must be at the ISE because the Child hasn't experienced that "bad feeling", yet. Unfortunately, this isn't necessarily true. The younger the age of the Child, the more compartmentalized feelings will be. As a result, it is possible for a Child to feel good/safe prior to an SSE.

If you assume you have found the ISE and proceed to clear the event, you may only get a temporary result. For this reason, it's best not to rely solely on this test. A more accurate test is to go immediately before the event and find out how the Child feels about *herself*. A Child can feel good at any given moment but may not necessarily love and accept herself. This is because feeling "good" and feeling "loved" are separate states.

If the Child loves and accepts herself, prior to the event playing out, it's a safe bet you have located the ISE.

This gives you four tests to help you zero in on the ISE.

1. Age Test
2. Feeling Test
3. Safety Test
4. Self-Acceptance Test

Step 8: Identify trapped feelings.

What feelings are still trapped in the event? Children lack the ability to experience mixed emotions. They compartmentalize their feelings. This means that one minute the Child can be feeling happy, the next minute they can be sad, then angry, then something else. This can make regressing into childhood events somewhat complicated because the feeling that led you back into an event may not be the causal feeling. For example, you Bridge back on a feeling of sadness, the client lands in an event, you begin the uncovering procedure only to find that the Child is feeling scared. You might be tempted to assume that you lost the Bridge. But there can be multiple feelings trapped in the same event.

If you move forward and back in the event, you may find that the feeling you Bridged back on is still there. For example, if the Child is feeling okay, instruct the client to go to the next significant feeling. You may find that the feeling is there. It's just been anchored to a specific moment in the event.

This baby-step approach helps to encourage revivification by validating the client's perceptions of what's happening. Once the client gains clarity about what's happening in the scene, you can invite them to just tell you the Story by asking, "What's happening? Tell me the Story as it's happening now."

Step 10: Identify decisions.

What decision(s) are being made? The subconscious mind's Prime Directive is to ensure survival. A survival program is a set of instructions, installed during the ISE, that says, "Whenever these conditions arise, respond by feeling/thinking/doing this (to avoid or minimize pain)." This programming comes out of the meanings assigned to the various perceptions at the Initial Sensitizing Event (ISE).

When something happens, it will make an impression on the Child. What does that make the Child think? What meaning is being assigned to that experience? These decisions form a lens through which life will be viewed, in future.

Thoughts generate feelings. The emotions generated by these thoughts will drive then behaviors and/or responses which often form as coping strategies. If the Child is feeling fear, find out what's happening to generate the fear. For example, "What's happening that you're feeling that scared feeling?"

The Child's answer will be either a perception or a thought. If the Child responds with a perception such as seeing, hearing, smelling, tasting or a sensation, ask, "What does that make you think?" The thought will be the cause of the feeling of fear.

For example, the Child says, "Mom's talking on the phone."

CH: "What does that make you think?"

Child: "I'm not important."

CH: "How does that make you feel?"

Better yet, use a Sentence Stem, "The *thought* 'I'm not important' makes me *feel* (put an ending on it.)" Thoughts become beliefs. Beliefs decide what we're going to get in life.

If the Child responds with a thought such as, "I'm going to die!" or "I'm not wanted", reality-check these thoughts with Adult Consciousness by asking Grownup, "Is that true? (Child) thinks that he's going to die." Of course, obviously, the Child isn't going to die. The Adult client is proof of this! But the subconscious mind doesn't know this. You can neutralize an irrational fear by informing the Child of the truth.

If Adult Consciousness verifies the perception of the Child as true, for example, "Mom didn't want another baby", the task then becomes one of helping the Child come to acceptance. Never change the facts, only the feelings.

Step 9: Uncover the layers.
The uncovering process occurs in layers. As you bring one aspect to conscious awareness, another aspect will often come to the surface. When you release a layer, often you'll find that there's a deeper layer beneath it. Some people call this "peeling the onion."

With every layer you release, access to a deeper layer of awareness is granted, allowing more detail to safely be brought to conscious awareness where it can be released and learned from. Remember, the devil is in the details!

What's the feeling?
The first level of perception will be the physical sensation. This is the Child's initial response to what's happening in the environment. Focus

on the feeling in the body. Does it feel comfortable or uncomfortable? Is that a good feeling or a bad feeling?

Tune in the five senses. What is the Child seeing? Hearing? Smelling? Tasting? Touching? How does that make them feel *in the body*?

What's the thought?
The second level of perception is cognition. This is the process of making sense of what's happening. The situation is being evaluated, based on how it feels. This forms an opinion which may or may not have any basis in truth. These opinions form the foundation of beliefs which make up the client's story. The problem is that children are very black and white in their thinking. What's happening is interpreted as either good or bad.

Children are also very absolute in their thinking. They readily believe that it will *always* be like this, and it will *never* end. Remember, the thoughts of the Child are not always based in truth or fact. Events are often misinterpreted. Over time, if left unchecked, erroneous thoughts can form false beliefs which generate uncomfortable emotional responses.

Because our beliefs tell us what to expect, and how to respond to circumstances in future, decisions made in childhood can be deciding what we get in life as adults. This is why we want to bring adult consciousness back into the event to re-evaluate the ISE. Adult consciousness has the maturity with which to reality-check the Child's interpretation of the experience.

What's the emotion?
The third level of perception is emotional. Emotions don't just happen. They come in response to our thoughts. This is the basis of

Thought-Cause-Alignment Theory. "The thought (X) makes me feel (Y)." In this way, every child learns how to respond to similar situations, should they arise in future.

When an emotional response seems irrational, it's because it's out of time. When seen as a response to the thoughts of the Inner Child, the response will be perfectly reasonable, based on subconscious logic. For example, a panic attack may seem like an irrational response. But when the thought behind that response is discovered to be, "I'm going to die!" the emotion of fear is perfectly logical.

Emotions want to move. That's what they do. E-Motion. Energy in motion. Uncomfortable emotions motivate us to take action to do something so that we can feel better. When an emotion wants to move, it creates internal tension which tends to feel bad or uncomfortable. This is a signal coming from the subconscious level of mind to let the conscious mind know that we need to move or change something. For example, fear motivates us to run to safety. Feelings and emotions are how the subconscious mind communicates with the conscious mind.

When it gets blocked from expression, it doesn't give up. It just finds another way to express. This can result in unwanted physical, mental, or emotional symptoms. This symptom of the subconscious mind striving for recognition is called the Symptom Imperative (SI).

Burying a feeling, locking it in a box, dissolving it away, erasing it or deleting it are surface techniques which attempt to override the subconscious mind's Symptom Imperative. Bad idea! When you're dealing with an emotional issue, these techniques do a bang-on job of reinforcing the conscious mind's strategy of *avoiding* the real problem. It's like saying, "That uncomfortable feeling inside of you is DANGEROUS. It's NOT SAFE for you to feel that feeling. So, let's escape to your Happy Place. Let's dig a hole, put that bad feeling in the hole, and cover it up with happy-happy."

Suppressing, repressing, rejecting, abandoning, or disowning Parts of the self will fail to resolve the problem because they *are* the problem. When an emotion feels bad, it's looking for a way out. The key to releasing the subconscious mind's need for symptom expression is to give the feeling permission to express.

Like every therapeutic technique, masking and avoidance strategies have their place. For example, you can use them to good effect to manage symptoms of pain; or as a preliminary technique to provide proof that change is possible; or as a polishing technique to reinforce changes that have occurred. But just as painting over the rust won't get rid of the rust, masking and avoiding symptoms will, at best, offer only temporary relief. They are ineffective strategies for achieving long-term results with emotional issues because they fail to address the root cause of the problem.

What's the response or behavior?

Behaviors and response should be viewed as resource states. They are learned responses, based on past experiences, that were originally meant to be helpful. The problem is that a two-year-old's response may be problematic in adulthood. For example, panicking at the sight of a dog can be embarrassing for an adult and may inhibit their ability to enjoy life fully. But the response is not the problem. It's a subconscious strategy that worked in the past to meet an important need in the past. For example, if the Child was bitten by a dog at age two, the need for safety is well-served by avoiding dogs.

Behind every behavior/response is an emotion. Uncomfortable emotions serve the positive purpose of motivating us to take action to meet our needs. In this case, the perception of threat (dog) generates the emotion of fear. Fear tells us to run to safety. Releasing the feeling trapped inside the event that caused it will allow the client to identify the unmet needs of the two-year-old. They can then identify a more appropriate response which will allow the Child to grow up feeling safe around dogs.

When we take action to meet our needs, it adds to the resources we have in our memory banks. As a result, we learn how to meet our needs in similar situations in future. This is called "resilience."

According to Psychology Today, "resilience is the psychological quality that allows some people to be knocked down by the adversities of life and come back at least as strong as before. Rather than letting difficulties, traumatic events, or failure overcome them and drain their resolve, highly resilient people find a way to change course, emotionally heal, and continue moving toward their goals."

Troubleshooting the Uncovering Process

Age-appropriate language?

Words such as depressed, upset, outraged, betrayed, disappointed, worthless, or stressed may be appropriate to what's happening in the event, but they are not the words of a child. If the client is using complex language to describe a feeling, recognize that you're speaking to the Adult Consciousness of the client. Keep the focus on the feelings of the Child.

Bad feeling?
Very young children often have trouble finding words to describe their feelings. All the Child knows is that it feels "bad." Locate the feeling in the body. Then, ask the Child, "If that bad feeling (in your tummy) could speak right now what would it say?" This can give you a sense of what the actual emotion might be.

Tense/Tight?
Infants lack an emotional vocabulary because their experience is more body centered. If the client has regressed to infancy, keep the focus on sensations in the body. For example, tight, tense, hurt, hot, stuck, cramping, ache, wanting to run/kick/cry, etc. are appropriate words to describe the emotional experience of an infant.

Where do they feel it?
If you're dealing with a very young Child, it's okay to relax the rules about naming the actual emotion. A Child's initial response to what's happening will always be physical sensations. These physical sensations are feelings that can be released, especially when they are targeted in the torso.

Tight, tense, crampy feelings in the throat, chest, or gut point to trapped emotional energies. Releasing "that feeling" will bring rapid relief from the discomfort allowing more clarity about what is happening in the scene to cause it.

To release the feeling, just keep the focus on what's happening in the body. Ask, "Where do you feel that feeling in your body?" Give the feeling permission to be there. Then, invite the Child to describe how "that feeling" is expressing. Allowing the feeling to express releases the feeling. As a result, the client will feel better.

"I don't know"?

When the Child says, "I don't know", this isn't necessarily a block to awareness. It may be a statement of truth. A pre-verbal Child may not have a word to describe what they're feeling. Ask the Child, "Where do you feel that 'I don't know' feeling in your body?"

Confused?

Children are often confused by the things that are happening around or to them. If the uncomfortable feeling is new to the Child, it will generate confusion. Confusion is a child's initial response to anything unlike love. What specifically feels unloving? That could be the problem calling for resolution. It may also indicate that you have located an ISE!

Client using past tense?

If the client starts using past-tense language, bring them back to re-experiencing the event by instructing the client to say, "Here I am . . ." Then, add something to it. For example, "Here I am . . . and I feel (put an ending on it)." Or, "Here I am, with Mom, inside, feeling scared."

Vague image?

If the aspects coming to awareness are vague, use baby steps to help bring the picture into focus. Remember, there's something in this event that the client's subconscious mind has been protecting the client from. The subconscious mind's primary purpose is survival. That experience was stored in memory to ensure the client would know how to respond to similar situations in future. If the situation in the past was perceived as a threat, it's still a threat. Uncovering the aspects incrementally will respect the client's need for safety.

Dark?

If the client's first impression is "nothing", "dark", or "floating", their subconscious mind may have taken them back into the womb. To test, say, "I'm going to ask you a kind of weird question. You don't think the answer, you *feel* the answer. Does it feel like you're inside or outside Mom?"

Troubleshooting Tips

Make sure your client is in somnambulism. Somnambulism facilitates revivification.

Remove unrealistic expectations before you begin the regression. Some clients expect to experience a 3-D visual experience. This isn't true for everyone. Memory is stored the way it was recorded. For example, the "first impression" might be a physical sensation, particularly if you Bridged back to an event in infancy.

Resistance can show up as thinking and analyzing. Recognize this as the conscious mind's attempt to control. To stay ahead of the conscious mind's tendency to try to control, work quickly!

The subconscious mind is the feeling mind. Teach the client to stay focused on the feeling. Instruct them to *feel* the answer to the question and to go with their first impression. For example, "Does it *feel* like it's daytime or nighttime?" "Does it *feel* like you're inside or outside?"

CHAPTER 8: RESISTANCE RESOLVED?

R*esistance does not mean that the client is being difficult. It's simply evidence that you don't yet have a Contract that allows that (whatever you're bumping into) to be a part of the process. You need both conscious and subconscious permission to guide the process.* ~ **The Devil's Therapy**

Resistance is the only problem you ever need to deal with in a regression hypnotherapy session. Resistance is not the problem. Resistance is simply fear. Fear is an emotion that arises in the face of a perceived threat. What is it? What is the client trying to avoid – consciously or unconsciously? What does the client not want to face? That's the real problem!

Resistance is a block to allowing the real problem to be brought to the surface of awareness where it can be healed. When you bump into resistance, realize that either the conscious mind or the subconscious mind does not want to go there. This should tell you that you're on the threshold of something important! Stay right where you are and work on uncovering the specific nature of the block – then release it!

The conscious mind is never fully out of the picture and when you get too close to emotional content it will try to block the process. This is why it's imperative, during the uncovering process, that the client answers quickly. It keeps the conscious, thinking mind out of the picture.

You need to work quickly to stay ahead of the conscious mind's tendency to step in and take control. Was your countback brisk and authoritative?

The first three uncovering questions serve to enhance revivification. This will allow the valuable details of the event to be made available for review and evaluation. If you skip over these critical questions, you'll likely lose your way.

If, on the other hand, you hold your client accountable for the results, and do not allow them to avoid (which is their learned coping strategy), you'll break through the seal on "forbidden memories."

The biggest mistake is to try to go beyond the client's threshold of readiness. For example, after following the Bridge, you begin the uncovering procedure by asking the client, "Daytime or nighttime?" and the client responds, "Nothing." Stop right there. The client isn't answering the question. The only available options are "daytime" or "nighttime". Either the client isn't regressing or there's a block to awareness. Whatever you do, do *not* proceed until the client answers the first uncovering question.

The moment the conscious mind steps in, it will do its best to block you. When that happens, deal with it! Remind the client that:

> 1) The only thing you care about is the feeling; the client's job is to stay focused on the feeling.

2) You want them to *feel* the answer to the question – not think.
3) It doesn't have to make sense. *Later* it will all make sense.
4) They're right where they need to be. "That feeling" has everything to do with the problem they've come to you for help in resolving.

Satisfy the conscious mind's need for logic and reason. This allows it to remain curious and observe what's being revealed through the process instead of being a backseat driver. Then, immediately, bring the focus of attention back to the feeling.

The Steps:

1. Find the feeling.
2. Validate the feeling.
3. Quantify the feeling.
4. Name the emotion.
5. Step into the event.

Step 1: Find the feeling.
Immediately check to see if the client is still connected to the Bridge by asking, "True or false – you feel the feeling?" If they're feeling the feeling, you're good to go!

The objective is to get the first question answered by gently greasing the hinges to allow more information to come to conscious awareness. If the client's answer to the question, ". . . you feel the feeling?" is "false", you've lost the Bridge. The question is *why?*

Step 2: Validate the feeling.
Continue to keep the focus on the feeling. "That feeling is allowed to be there. It has everything to do with (the presenting problem). Is that a good feeling or a bad feeling? (Comfortable or uncomfortable?)"

Step 3: Quantify the feeling.
Take a SUD. For example, "How strong is that uncomfortable feeling (in your tummy)?" (Amplify, if needed.) Remember, you need a strong Bridge to make it back to the ISE.

Remember, "that feeling" is a signal coming out of the ISE. If necessary, increase the client's connection to the awareness of "that feeling" by amplifying the feeling. For example, "Good! Focus on that feeling. Where in your body do you feel that feeling? Describe it to me. (Does it have a shape? A color? How big might "that feeling" be? Etc.)"

Step 4: Name the emotion.
"As you're feeling that (tight) feeling in your (tummy), what *emotion* might "that feeling" be – sad, mad, glad, scared or something else?"

Step 5: Step into the event.
"As you're feeling that (scared) feeling in your (gut) . . . become aware . . . does it *feel* like it's daytime or nighttime where your mind now has you? First impression." Once the client answers this question, you're in! Immediately go to the next uncovering question. "Good! As you're feeling that (scared) feeling (in your gut), does it *feel* like you're inside or outside? First sense."

Troubleshooting Resistance

Vague responses?

If the client's responses during the uncovering procedure are vague, check to make sure the client is still feeling the feeling. The stronger the emotion, the deeper the hypnosis. Take a SUD.

If the client has lost the connection to the feeling, go back to where you can find the feeling, bring it up powerfully, and Bridge back on it.

Remember, revivification requires somnambulism. Is the client in a state of somnambulism? Conduct a test for state.

Is the client trying to remember? If so, the conscious mind is blocking the process. The only thing you're interested in is the client's first impression. Give the suggestion, "Don't think. *Feel* the answer to the questions. The only thing that matters is how it feels."

Client is using past tense?

If the client is speaking in past tense, you're speaking to the conscious mind. This could be an avoidance strategy or the client could be consciously remembering the event. In either case, you need the conscious mind to step aside. Say, "I'll get to you in a moment, Grownup. Right now, I need you to stay in the background while I speak to (Child)." Then, rewind the event, instruct the client to use present tense language, and replay the event. For example, "In a moment, I'm going to count from three down to one. On the count of one, it's happening all over, again. 3, 2, 1. Be there. Tell me everything as it's happening, now. Say, 'Here I am . . . and I feel (put an ending on it.)"

Continue with the uncovering procedure. For example: "What's happening as (you're sitting in the chair)?"

To keep the client in the scene, ask, "What's happening *now*?"

To move to the next important moment, ask, "What happens *next*?"

Once you have a sense of what's happening in the scene, ask, "What does that make you *think*, (Child)?"

Remember, the underlying problem is not the feeling and it's not what happened. It's how the Child was interpreting what was happening and how that made them feel. To identify the cause of the problem, find the thought that creates a spike of emotion.

If the client reports feeling insecure, stressed, or inadequate, they're giving you a thought. To identify the underlying emotion, use a Stem. For example, "Repeat after me and put an ending on it. 'The thought *insecure* make me feel . . . (put an ending on it)." Then, "Where do you feel that (sad) feeling in your body? How young might you be that you're feeling (sad)?"

Nothing 'bad' is happening?

If you're Bridging back on an uncomfortable feeling like fear, anger or sadness, and the client goes back to a happy event, poke around a little. Sometimes, you'll discover that the event started out as a happy experience, then something happened to change that. The 'bad' feeling is still trapped in the event. You just need to find it.

If the event doesn't seem to be revealing too much, give the instruction to "move to the next significant moment that has everything to do with that (sad) feeling."

If you still can't find the 'bad' feeling, it's possible that the client is trying to avoid a painful event. In this case, you have lost the Bridge. Repeat the process of provoking the feeling for Affect Bridge.

Slow or No Response?

If you regress the client into a past event and begin the uncovering procedure only to find the client's answers to the uncovering question are slow, wait a few moments, then ask, "True or False, you're aware of where your mind has you?" Often, the client will have a sense of where they have "landed" but may be trying to figure things out. In this case, instruct the client to answer with their first impression. Remind them that it doesn't have to make sense.

If the client says that they don't know where they're at, respond matter-of-factly, "I *know* you don't know. Just give me your first impression. Reality has nothing to do with it. Pretend you know! (while lightly tapping on the client's forehead) One, two, three. First impression. Daytime or nighttime?"[24]

Client Can't See?

Keep the focus of attention on sensory input. That's the first impression regarding what's happening in the event. Say, "Seeing is over-rated. Use your other senses – hearing, sensing, feeling. What's your first sense? Your first impression?"

If the client is unaware or can't see, say, "There's a reason for that. Your mind doesn't want you to see." Then, speak directly to the subconscious mind, "You're here. There's nothing to protect her from. I ask you to understand that whatever is back there, whatever you are protecting this person from, she survived it at least once. We

---

[24] If you're working online, substitute finger snaps for the forehead tap.

have proof of that because she's alive in this office today. It couldn't have been that bad. I suggest to you that this is the perfect place and time to get her healed of this condition. I ask you, subconscious mind, to allow (Client) to have all the information stored on this scene, situation, or event."

Alternately, you can have the client ask their own subconscious mind. For example, "Subconscious, I can handle it. Let me have the information so I can heal!" Then give the command, "At the count of 3, (she's) going to feel those emotions. I ask you to let (her) feel those emotions. One, there's the feelings. Two, trapped so deep inside, now welling forth. And on the next count, there they are, as real as you've ever allowed her to feel them before. And three, there's the feeling. (Client), give me a word, describe that feeling."

Continue bridging back to the ISE.

Client can't hear?

Not being able to hear is common when the client goes to the womb. In this case, the Child is aware, but sounds will be muffled. Sometimes, there's something happening that the Child doesn't *want* to hear. In either case, you can turn up the volume by saying, "In a moment I'm going to snap my fingers three times. As I do, in this situation where your mind has you, it will be as if *the volume goes up*, and you hear everything being said in this moment. I'll sit quietly and wait for your report. When you know what's being said, give me your report." (Snap, snap, snap!)

Client is apprehensive to face what's happening?

Ask the client, "True or false, you're aware of where your mind has you?"

If the client is aware of where they're at, chunk down to specific sensory input. Tease out the aspects incrementally. For example, what does the client hear? Smell? Taste? Sense? Know?

Lack of emotion?
This requires some care. If the client's coping strategy is to stay in their head to avoid feelings, their grownup mind may be stepping in to prevent the emotions from coming to awareness. The subconscious mind will always protect the Child. Child Parts are feeling Parts. If "that feeling" threatens to overwhelm the Child, the subconscious mind will block it.

Focus on what's happening in the body. Ask, "Does it seem like it's too much?" Remember, safety is Law #1. If it seems like it's too much, you can provide safety by placing the Child in background and continue the uncovering work by having the grownup give you a report. Because the Adult and Child share the same feelings, the client knows what the Child is feeling.

You just need to get a general idea about what's happening in the event before testing for the ISE. Ask Grownup, "What's happening? Who is there? What feelings is the Child feeling?"

If the lack of emotion is coming out of the client's younger self, this is evidence of a big pocket of emotional energy with a lid on it. Bridge back to "the first time it just wasn't worth feeling, when *not*-feeling was a good idea."

Client is racing through the event?
Racing through an event is evidence that the client is feeling overwhelmed. Chunk down and bring the focus back to the feeling in the body. Then, releasing some of the internal stress. This will help

to improve cognitive ability allowing you to continue the uncovering work. Remember, the causal event is seldom a high-intensity experience. Keep the focus on "that feeling" and continue Bridging back until you find the ISE. Resolving the ISE will weaken the intensity of emotions trapped in Subsequent Sensitizing Events (SSEs).

Child is feeling confused or overwhelmed?
Confusion is often the first response to a distressing situation in infancy and can indicate that you have found the ISE. If the client has regressed to a young age and reports feeling confused or overwhelmed, say, "You're right where you need to be. Your subconscious mind knows why you're here. You're ready for a breakthrough. Let this be your miracle moment and focus on that feeling."

Not having enough choices or enough information to be able to make sense of what's happening will generate anxiety in the Child. This indicates an unmet need which can find expression, later in life, as impatience or procrastination. When something is perceived to be either "too much" or "too little", it generates stress. For example, too much (or too little) information or choices, puts the mind into overload. As a result, the Child can't think. This can result in the Child deciding, "I'm not smart enough."

Client can't speak?
Inability to speak happens when the rational, logical part of the brain goes offline. Ask, "Does it feel like it's too much?" If so, a dissociative technique can provide much-needed safety. For example, you can guide the client to float up above the timeline and view the event from a higher perspective. Alternately, you can put the Child safely in the background and let the Adult tell you what's happening in the event.

Client says, "I'm stuck"?

"Stuck" is another way of saying, "I can't reason my way out of this." Check to see if you're still talking to the Child by asking, "True or false, you feel the feeling?" If the client is experiencing an emotion, you're talking to the Child. Bring awareness to "that stuck feeling" in the body and guide the client to name the emotion.

Child is experiencing physical pain?

Situations of abuse may have resulted in physical pain for the Child. Desensitizing physical pain can allow the client to continue with the uncovering procedure. For example, "Tend to your breathing and the *discomfort goes away* as you become aware of all that's happening to you. What's happening?"

While regression hypnotherapy does not change what happened in a past event, the client does not need to re-experience *physical* pain to heal. You just need to uncover enough about what happened to resolve the cause of the client's presenting issue.

Client reports gut-wrenching emotion or nausea?

Emotional pain can be converted into physical pain. For example, intense sensations in the gut such as cramping and nausea. Do not emerge the client from hypnosis. Instruct them to open their eyes and sit up. Remember, the client is still in a heightened state of suggestibility. Keep pouring the suggestions in. Give them a waste basket or bucket[25] and tell them to, "Get it out! The only place that feeling can hurt you is trapped inside! You get that out, you're going to feel so good!"

---

[25] I have never had a client vomit but several have gagged and spit up phlegm.

Once the client is stabilized, give them a drink of water. Check to see if they need to go to bathroom to refresh. When they return, ask, "Ready to go?" With the client's permission, return to the scene by saying, "Close your eyes. I'm going to count from three down to one. On the count of one, you're right back where you began."

Client starts coughing?

Any physical symptom is subconscious communicating in code. Coughing is code for something that needs to be expressed. Suggest, "That bark is code for what needs to be said. It all comes out when I snap my fingers (snap-snap-snap). That bark now turns to words. *You're allowed to say it.* Find the words now."

Client is shocked by what is revealed?

If the client is shocked or expresses disbelief by what is being revealed by their subconscious mind, *rewind and replay* the event for the purpose of gaining understanding. For example, "The whole scene rewinds and it all plays out, once again. Only this time, everything you've learned comes together in an understanding so that nothing comes as a surprise to you. It all becomes clear to you as your mind puts it all together. Three, two, one!"

Client abreacts?

During the uncovering procedure, memories seldom come flooding into conscious awareness all at once. Most of the time, it's a process of teasing out the information needed to release the underlying cause of the problem. This is because the subconscious mind doesn't recognize that the client isn't a Child, anymore. As far as it's concerned, that event is still a threat. We learn from a very early age to put a lid on our feelings. If the event was too overwhelming for the client, the first time, *it still is.*

When a feeling gets trapped inside it generates emotional and/or physical pain. All those unresolved thoughts and emotions are looking for a way out. When the pressure gets to be too much, they can find their way to the surface of consciousness, unexpectedly. That's when you'll get an abreaction. It happens. It's nothing to be afraid of. You just need to control it. The problem is that you can't cap an oil well when it's a geyser. What you *can* do is slow things down. Slowing things down will allow the client to take one perception, one thought, or one emotion at a time.

When the client lands in an event that immediately presents strong affect, there's no need to continue with the preliminary uncovering questions (daytime/nighttime, inside/outside). The client is well-aware of what's happening. What they need is sufficient safety to be able to face what's there. The easiest way to provide safety is to take charge of the process. Guide the client to step into the scene. Then, use autosuggestion to facilitate the uncovering process. Speaking out loud helps to release some of the pent-up emotional charge while keeping the client focused on what's happening in the event. For example: "3, 2, 1 … (client begins abreacting) 'Say, Here I am / And I feel (put an ending on it).'"

Realize that the client's subconscious mind is bringing you into this scene/event for a reason. There's a big pocket of pain trapped in this event and the subconscious mind is trusting you to give it some relief. This is good news! Prove that you can help by releasing the emotional charge and it will show you where the problem got started. Once you find the event, give the feeling permission to be there. Then, go straight into the releasing process. For example,

Client: "Scared! I feel scared!"

CH: "Where do you feel that scared feeling in your body?"

Client: (clutching gut)

CH: "Let me help you. That feeling is allowed to be there." (Proceed to guide the client to release the feeling, then validate any shift toward the better.)

Remember to validate every change for the better. Bringing the overall intensity down will give you access to more of the details. You don't have to completely neutralize the event. Just restore a sense of balance and control. If you're in a SSE, reassure the subconscious mind that you will come back to this event and take care of it. Then, ask permission to go back to take care of the cause of the problem so that you can Bridge back to the ISE.

Most of the time, going "upstream" to resolve the ISE will reduce the overall emotional charge feeding into subsequent events. As a result, when you return to the SSE, all that will be left, if anything, will be residual aspects. Just remember to keep your promise and return to the SSE after you have cleared the ISE!

Client is flooded with intense fear/terror?

Emotional intensity indicates you're right where the client's healing lies. But safety is the subconscious mind's Prime Directive. If the client is feeling overwhelmed by fear or terror, and you don't know what to do - *get them out*. They do not need to relive an event of terror. To get them out of the scene, give the suggestion, "Let the scene fade and grow peaceful with your breathing."

Wait for the client to stabilize. Then, say, "That's good. And go deeper." Give the client a few minutes to talk about what just happened. Listening provides safety while allowing the client to process that frightening experience. Listen first – then speak to provide the conscious mind with reason. For example, "When we're little, and we feel things we don't know how to feel, our tendency is to block ourselves off. That's how the mind works to protect us sometimes."

Pause a moment to let the suggestion sink in. Then, prepare the client to go back and process the event. For example, "Now, in a moment, we're going to go back to that scene. You know you're here with me, now. You're a grownup. You know there's nothing there that you haven't already lived through. Understand?"

Then set up for the releasing work. For example, "This time you are going to get the rest of those emotions out. The only place they can hurt you is trapped inside. You are always in control, but you *like* the thought of getting them out. This is where your healing lies. It feels so good to learn from the past without having to hide from it."

Use a directed regression back to the event, then test. For example, "3, 2, 1 – Be there. True or false, your mind has you in the same place it had you moments ago?"

If you get stuck or the dialogue process seems to stall, don't start asking questions. It's too soon for that. Instead, echo back what the Part just told you as a question, or rephrase what the Part just told you. Then, add those three magic words, "Tell me more."

~ **Dream Healing Practitioner Guidebook:** *A Healer's Guide to Uncovering the Secret Messages of Your Dreams*

CHAPTER 9:
GOT EVERYTHING?

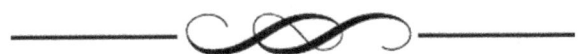

T*he causal event is like an infected, open wound. What makes it so painful is that the toxic emotions trapped inside the event create internal pressure. Releasing the trapped emotions relieves internal pressure, which brings the client relief. Release everything and the energy trapped in the event of wounding can be directed toward healing.* – **The Devil's Therapy**

The reason the client hasn't been able to have what they want (their stated therapeutic goal) is because there are unconscious blocks preventing them from having that experience. As you release these internal blocks, the client will begin to experience greater clarity from which to make better choices that support health and well-being. The key to getting a complete resolution of the client's issue is to release everything that has been getting in their way.

When you give the subconscious mind permission to express what it feels to be true, the client will experience an immediate sense of relief. For example, releasing brings mental clarity by undoing false beliefs. Clarity restores the power of choice which brings empowerment that is based on subconscious truth.

The subconscious mind is the Child mind. Uncomfortable feelings are just how Child Parts let the conscious mind know that there's a problem calling for resolution. Releasing internal blocks restores balance and harmony to the mind-body system because our natural state is one of well-being.

There are many ways to encourage emotional release, including speaking out loud (expressing thoughts), emoting (expressing emotions), and physical movement (taking action to move the energy out; for example, striking a pillow). The most used emotional-release techniques in regression hypnotherapy are talking, tapping, and Pillow Therapy.

Talking

Simply allowing the client to talk about their feelings can bring a measure of relief. Add autosuggestion and you have a much more powerful technique than direct suggestion.

Remember, regression hypnotherapy is an interactive process. For example, Parts Work occurs during the transformational phase of the healing process. You're having a conversation with Parts of the client. Child Parts are feeling Parts. Give the Part permission to speak! Remember, everything that comes out of the client's mouth is a suggestion they are giving themselves. If the client says, "I feel scared", that's a statement of truth.

There doesn't have to be a reason for that feeling. The subconscious truth *is* the feeling. But when there doesn't seem to be a reason for the feeling, the client will blame themselves for feeling "bad." You can use the EFT setup phrase to make it safe for the client to allow more of the uncomfortable feeling. For example, "Even though I feel scared,

I deeply and completely accept myself." This allows the feeling to be there while removing any self-blame. Continuing to focus on the feeling will make it stronger. Inviting the client to say, "I'm allowed to feel (scared)" will reduce resistance because acceptance of a feeling makes it safe to allow the feeling to be there.

Tapping

If you don't know tapping techniques, you can simply have the client tap on the Karate Chop Point while guiding them through the autosuggestion process. Tapping and talking, while focusing on a significant feeling that is expressing in the body has the added benefit of having a Confusional effect which can help to deepen the hypnosis.[26]

The way to release an uncomfortable feeling is to feel the feeling *fully*. The problem is that those feelings don't feel good. As the subconscious mind's Prime Directive is safety, your priority is to make it safe for your client to *allow* uncomfortable feelings and emotions to be part of the process. This begins by teaching your clients how to feel better by releasing uncomfortable feelings.

The Steps:

1. Acknowledge the feeling.
2. Accept the feeling.
3. Allow the feeling.

---

[26] You'll find information about common reversals in Ready for Regression: Hypnosis Practitioner's Guide to Preparing Clients for Effective Regression Hypnotherapy

Step 1: Acknowledge the feeling

Begin by establishing a series of truisms. This will help increase compliance. For example: "There's a feeling inside that I just don't like/ I've tried running from it / I've tried shoving it down / putting a lid on it / numbing and swallowing it away / That hasn't worked/ I can still feel it!"

Step 2: Accept the feeling

Next, guide the client to take ownership of the feeling. This will help to establish a preliminary agreement to allow the feeling. "I'm allowed to feel it / because this is *my feeling* / and if I can feel it, I can heal it / I'm allowed to feel it / And I'm allowed to release it / so I can feel better."

Step 3: Allow the feeling

After acknowledging and accepting the feeling, the final step is to test for compliance. With sufficient reason, the client will agree to cooperate and give permission for the feeling to come up. For example: "As I speak, that feeling is coming up inside of me." Then deliver the following question as a suggestion, "True or false – you feel the feeling."

If the feeling is present, you have successfully tested for compliance. Suggestions can then be offered to validate and amplify the feeling.

If the feeling is *not* present, the following suggestions will further address the reversal. For example: "Even though there are Parts of me that might try to think or avoid / I'm allowed to feel my feelings/ this is the perfect place / I'm allowed to feel *all* my feelings / even the bad ones / because all my feelings are good / they're there to help and guide me / so I can heal / so I accept this feeling."

If you have identified a specific objection to allowing the feeling, you can address it here. Otherwise, "it's not safe" is generally a good starting place. Most often the client will nod in agreement as they say the words, "It's not safe." For example: "Even though *it's not safe* to feel this feeling / I choose to let it come up strong within me / so I can heal / because I deeply and completely accept this feeling / And if I can feel it / I can heal it."

Statements of choice help to empower the client and encourage greater compliance. If you follow a statement of truth with a statement of choice based in reason, it will satisfy the conscious mind's need for control, making it more reasonable to allow the feeling to come up to conscious awareness. For example: "Even though *it's not safe* to feel this feeling / I let myself go where I need to go / see what I need to see / hear what I need to hear / and feel what I need to feel / so I can feel better / because I deeply and completely accept myself."

Notice how this is setting up for regression? "Even though *it's not safe* to feel this feeling / I do what I need to do to heal / because nothing else has worked / And I deeply and completely accept myself, anyway. / And even though I don't *want to feel this feeling* / I can feel it / I feel it in my body … "

Repeat the compliance test, here, "Where in your body do you *feel it?*"

Pillow Therapy

Tapping is effective for releasing most emotions. But when it comes to the really big, hairy-scary feelings, a pillow is more effective. The larger movements of Pillow Therapy can quickly discharge the uncomfortable energies trapped in the nervous system of the body.

You need a sturdy pillow for Pillow Therapy. The firmer, the better. Pillows stuffed with poly-fill are too soft and mushy. They tend to slime around. You need a solid, firm pillow that can absorb the impact of releasing intense emotions. The bigger the pillow, the better. This gives the client a nice big target area to hit. It also makes it safer for the client by ensuring that they won't hurt themselves if they really let loose.

In addition to your large, firm pillow, keeping a futon bolster on hand for your "heavy hitters" can be very useful. Because a futon is very heavy and dense, it can really take a beating, and the bolster is the perfect shape to slip between the client's legs, holding it securely in place.

Before initiating Pillow Therapy, make sure that your clients understand they're not hitting or punching the pillow. Hitting and punching can generate resistance because it's aggressive. Pillow Therapy is about *releasing* the energy that's responsible for causing the client pressure and pain. Make it clear to the client that what you're asking them to do is *pump* the uncomfortable feeling out of the body and into the pillow. You're giving the feeling a way out by giving it a place to go – into the pillow. This gives the client a way to safely discharge the energy that's been trapped inside. As a result, they will feel better, often surprisingly quickly.

Baseball Bat

If your client has arthritis or shoulder issues, they're going to have difficulty releasing into the pillow because they're too stiff to be able to get those big movements that really help to move the feelings out. Often, they're afraid that they're going to hurt themselves. As a result, they'll hold back.

The solution is to give the client a plastic baseball bat[27]. This provides leverage to allow the bigger movement. It also makes a very satisfying "thwack" sound when it comes into contact with the pillow.

Tennis Ball
If your client has really long fingernails, when she makes a fist and starts pumping the feeling into the pillow, her nails are going to dig into the palms of her hands. When a person is focused on feeling strong emotions, they're in *deep* hypnosis. This produces analgesia.

A client in somnambulism won't notice that she's bleeding all over your pillow. The solution is to keep a racquet ball or a tennis ball in your office. When it comes time to do the releasing work, place the tennis ball into the palm of the client's hand and tell her to make a fist around the ball. Then, place their fist into the pillow.

Pump the client's arm up and down a few times as you give the suggestion to "get it out." The ball will protect the client's hands when they start releasing the energy into the pillow. It will also save you having to launder your pillow!

Puke Bucket
Some clients can release some pretty nasty stuff. That's good. But if the client feels like they were going to vomit, (it's rare but it happens) having a large bowl or small bucket that you can place in the client's lap can make the difference between holding onto the feeling and getting it out. Get it out and let it go!

---

[27] A Nerf bat works well, too.

The Steps:

1. Find the feeling.
2. Verify good feeling/bad feeling.
3. Offer a choice.
4. Grind down to the emotion.
5. Validate change.

Step 1: Find the feeling.

The releasing process begins with finding the feeling in the body and naming it. Ultimately, you want the client to name the *emotion* and give it permission to express. But at the beginning of the healing process, this isn't critical. It's more important that the client learn to allow feelings to come to awareness. Regression hypnotherapy is, after all, a learning process.

Being client-centered means working with whatever the client gives you, not demanding that the client get it right the first time. It is okay to start the releasing process by working with a 'betrayed,' 'worthless,' or 'stupid' feeling. Using the client's own words will help to increase rapport. Just keep the focus on the body. For example, "Where in the body do you feel that 'worthless feeling'?"

Locate the feeling in the body. That's the feeling the conscious mind doesn't like and wants to get rid of it. What the client is experiencing in the body is direct subconscious communication. It's a signal coming out of the event that caused it.

Teach your clients to accept and honor their feelings by validating whatever they are experiencing in the body. "That feeling" is a Child Part speaking.

Step 2: Verify good feeling/bad feeling.
Children are taught that it's wrong to feel certain feelings. They're taught that some feelings are bad. As a result, when the Child feels "that feeling", they interpret it to mean that *they* are bad. This disconnects them from their intrinsic goodness and worth.

When the client finds the feeling in the body, ask, "Is that a "good" feeling or a "bad" feeling?" This is inviting the Child to step forward and be heard. Remind the client that it's okay to feel their feelings. Let them take ownership of their feelings. For example, "This is *your feeling*. You're allowed to feel all your feelings."

Remember, the subconscious mind is the conscious mind *of the past*. Children are black and white thinkers. Either it feels good or it feels bad. That's all you need to know to get started.

Step 3: Offer A choice.
A permission-based approach helps to satisfy the primary needs of both the conscious and subconscious Mind. The subconscious mind needs safety. The conscious mind needs to be in control. Offering a choice satisfies both these needs.

Once the client is focused on that "bad feeling" in the body, ask, "Do you want to *hold onto* that feeling . . . or *release it* so you can feel better?" With the client's consent, you are ready to begin releasing the feeling. The goal is not to get rid of the feeling. The feeling isn't bad. It just *feels* bad because it's trapped inside, generating pressure. The goal is to give the feeling a way out so that the client can feel better.

Step 4: Grind down to the emotion.
Clients will often use words like "anxious", "stressed", "upset", "worthless", etc. to describe how they're feeling. Recognize that these

words are labels which allow the client to get some emotional distance from the actual emotion. "Scared" or "angry" are emotions that can be released so you need to grind down to the actual emotion.

Keep the focus on "that feeling in the body." The more specific the client can be in describing what they are experiencing, the more complete the release will be. For example, a general term like "anxiety," or "upset," will be less effective than, "This scared, tight, tense knot in my gut" or, 'This anger stuck in my throat."

If the client says, "I feel anxious, bad, upset, stressed; rejected, betrayed or inadequate," or, "I feel like I don't belong," or "I'm not wanted," begin the releasing process on the thought. For example, "the thought 'I don't belong'" or "the thought 'I'm not wanted'". Releasing "that (worthless) feeling in the (gut)" or "that (I'm not wanted) feeling in the (heart) will allow the feeling to move. As a result, it will begin to change.

Some clients speak in metaphors. For example, "I feel like there's a heavy weight" or "I feel like I can't breathe." Use it. You can get good results working with the imagery suggested by the metaphor because the native language of the subconscious mind is symbolic. For example, "The thought 'this heavy weight' makes me feel (put an ending on it)" or "The thought 'I can't breathe' makes me feel . . . (put an ending on it.)"

Whenever possible, pair the thought and associated sensation together. For example, "The thought (betrayed) *makes me feel* (angry.)" Or, "The thought (unworthy) *makes me feel* this (tight knot in my gut)[28]."

---

[28] Matt Sison

This will help the client make the distinction between thinking and feeling. As a result, the use of emotional words will become more natural and frequent.

If the client gives you another thought, say, "Give me another word. What's another word for that feeling?" In this way, you can grind down to an emotion such as sad, scared or angry.

If the client seems to be dancing around the emotional word, ask directly, "What *emotion* might that be?"

Better yet, offer a multiple-choice option. For example, "What emotion might that be – mad, sad, glad, angry, scared or something else?" This helps to improve emotional literacy.

Keep the focus on the body. When the client can identify the emotion, give the instruction to focus on "that (scared, mad, sad, lonely, or hurt) feeling and notice how it feels in the body." Releasing both the named emotion and how it's expressing in the body at the same time will get you a quicker, more complete, release of the patterned response.

Step 5. Validate change.
Releasing often results in insights bubbling up to conscious awareness. When this happens, acknowledge it! When a client has released something, or experiences an insight say, "Good job!" or "Well done!" These two words are powerfully validating and encourage the client to continue with the process. Remember, emotional energies trapped inside generate internal stress, and stress inhibits cognition. Releasing trapped emotional energies will result in greater mental clarity for the client which can make the uncovering procedure much easier for you.

In addition, every insight or shift toward a better feeling can be used as evidence that change is occurring. The problem is that change tends not to happen all at once. You need to bring the client's attention to the fact that change is occurring and that what they are doing is working. This encourages the subconscious mind to integrate all changes while making it safe to allow more emotional stuff to be brought to the surface where it can be cleared.

If the client has experienced an emotional release, give them a moment to rest and notice the better feeling. Help the client to realize that something has happened by bringing attention to the shift toward the better, no matter how small. For example, if the client reports feeling more relaxed, more peaceful, or more safe and secure, say, "Notice how much better you feel. You're allowed to feel better. Just take a moment, now, to let all these good feelings become a part of you now."

Contrasting an uncomfortable feeling, which the client was feeling just a moment ago, with how much better the client feels *now*, can help the client to recognize that what you're doing is working. For example: "A moment ago you were feeling (all those uncomfortable feelings). Notice how much better you feel *now*. Feeling a feeling releases the feeling. You let yourself feel it to release it. Good job! Notice how much better you feel for having released it. Your (gut) feels better. Something has changed. You're changing! You're allowed to change and let all your good feelings flow back into you."

If the client experiences an insight, validate it! A new sense of order is being established at a subconscious level of mind. What have they just discovered? What are they learning? Help the client realize that *they* are changing.

Troubleshooting the Releasing Process

Regress or Release?

Your best overall strategy is to deal with whatever the client gives you. If there's lots of energy trapped in a SSE, don't shoot for the ISE. Stay there and release some of the internal pressure. The objective is to drain the swamp. But sometimes, you have to deal with the alligators first. Releasing the client's resistance to facing their feelings will help to restore clarity, clearing the path to the ISE.

Clearing a few SSE's can produce insights. These insights can then be transferred into the ISE and used to transform the cause of the client's issue. And because the subconscious mind tends to generalize all learning, releasing a significant emotional charge that's been trapped in an SSE can have a backwash effect into the ISE, weakening or even neutralizing it completely.

While finding the roots of the problem in childhood can help you to get quicker results, the client must have sufficient clarity with which to make sense of what happened in the ISE. Taking the time to clear an emotionally-charged SSE can give you a client who is better-equipped to face the truth of a traumatic childhood. They will also be better able to discover the connection between past experiences and the presenting symptoms.

If the client lands in a pocket of intense emotions that's overwhelming their senses, you can rewind to move them to before the intensity comes on. Take the client to a point prior to the overwhelm where they're still feeling safe. You can then prepare them for what's "going to happen." This gets the client out of the overwhelm without having to get them out of the event. You can then release any apprehension about "what's going to happen".

If the client has released an emotional block, rewind and replay the portion of the event to test and make sure the feeling is completely released. As the client's emotional energies come back into balance, they'll have greater clarity with which to report. As a result, more detail will be made available which can lead to insights.

Big hairy-scary event?
The problem with a traumatic memory is that, often, there's too much happening, all at once. It's all happening much too quickly, and the Child just wasn't prepared for it. What happened took them by surprise. And they didn't have the resources needed to handle it.

If the client gets flooded with too much emotional energy, or too much information, you don't have to get them out of the event. Just say, "Everything stops." Freeze-framing the event provides safety which will allow you to uncover and release the cause of the client feeling overwhelmed.

If what's happening is too much for the client, take them after "what just happened" and process the event in hindsight. Fast-forward past all the high-intensity drama to *after* the event is over and release the feelings associated with the story using past-tense language.

The objective for releasing immediately after the event is to neutralize the negative impact. This allows the mind to process the event as finished. It then integrates the memory as a past event. This is supported by research which shows that when support is provided immediately *after* a traumatic experience occurs there doesn't have to be any lasting effects.

When a person has a chance to process their thoughts and feelings immediately following a traumatic experience, they can release the emotional charge. That's what keeps a person stuck in an event from the past.

Once the subconscious mind realizes that the event is over, it will start to relax. When that happens, you can guide the client to immediately *before* the event to prepare the Child for "what's going to happen" by providing the most important information – the Child is going to survive! Not only is Grownup living proof of this, but *this time*, the Child doesn't have to go through it alone.

Need more detail?

Sometimes, the client will try to race through an event. The problem is that they're skipping over all the details. You need those details to get a complete resolution of the problem. You can prevent this avoidance strategy by instructing the client to "pause" the event. You can then deal with one thing at a time by titrating the event.

Titrating is a method of chunking down to make what's happening in an event more manageable. If the client is feeling overwhelmed, instead of trying to deal with everything all at once, you can segment the event and work on one piece at a time. Start with the beginning of the story. What's the first perception, thought, or feeling that causes an emotional spike? Focus on that. Release it. Help the client experience some relief before moving onto the next aspect.

For example,

- The look on her face makes me feel . . .
- The sound of his voice makes me feel . . .
- The thought "I'm not wanted" makes me feel . . .

- The smell of booze on his breath makes me feel . . .
- Feeling stuck, no way out makes me feel . . .
- The thought, "I can't breathe!" makes me feel. . .
- This tightness in my chest makes me think . . .
- This knot in my gut makes me think . . .
- This pounding in my heart makes me think . . .
- This fear/ anger / sadness (in my gut/chest/throat)

Segmenting, in this way, is a baby-steps approach that allows you to slow things down, making it safer for the client to face their own thoughts and feelings. This helps to build confidence in the client as they discover they can face what happened and do the work necessary to heal themselves.

Did something change? Validate it!

The word 'validation' comes from the Latin verb *valere* which means "to be strong or true." The words valid and valor share the same root. Validation literally means "to make strong" or "to declare as valid [true]." Another meaning is "to substantiate" - that is, to verify and mark as substantial. That's what you want to do. Whenever there's a shift toward a better feeling, bring the client's attention to it.

Most of the time, healing doesn't happen all at once. It's a process of accruing the benefits, one release at a time. To encourage the client to allow more releases to occur, give the client permission to "rest and relax for a moment" following each significant release. Let the client realize something has shifted because they may not always notice it.

Following a round of releasing, instruct the client to go inside and notice what, if anything, has changed. If the client doesn't volunteer any specific information, ask, "Do you feel the same, worse or better?"

The answer to this question will tell you what the next step needs to be. It's a test.

Client feels lightheaded?
Light-headedness is often a result of hyperventilating. Slow things down. Encourage the client to breathe deeper. Offer them a sip of water. Give them a moment to rest and recalibrate before continuing.

Client takes a deep breath?
Something has just shifted. Pause for a moment to acknowledge this and notice what's changed. Say, "Notice the space you have just created." Then, give the client a moment to soak up the transformation.

Client feels better?
If the client feels *better*, use autosuggestion to validate the better feeling. For example, have the client say, "I feel better." This is a statement of truth. As such, it validates next autosuggestion, "I'm allowed to feel better." This pairing of a statement of truth (I feel better) with a statement of permission (I'm allowed to feel better) will encourage more feelings to come to the surface to be released.

Client feels the same?
Releasing techniques work. When what you're doing doesn't seem to be working, there's always a reason. If the intensity of a feeling isn't coming down, either there's pressure pushing up into the event from an earlier event, or you need to be more specific to target the real problem.

If you're too general, you'll get nowhere. Are you being specific enough?

Is the client tuned into feeling the feeling in the body? Are they tuned into the problem? To release it, the client needs to be *in it*, experiencing the feeling fully.

Is the client still feeling the same emotion or is it something different? This is the most common reason for a SUD level going up. When the client releases the aspect that they were focused on, the subconscious mind will automatically push whatever was beneath that feeling to the surface. The client won't realize this, however, because they still feel 'bad'.

Releasing creates a void. As a result, following an emotional release, another uncomfortable feeling may rush to the surface of awareness to be healed. The problem is that the client doesn't know this. All he knows is that he's still feeling uncomfortable. Because the emerging feeling is uncomfortable, the client may report feeling the same or worse when, in fact, the original feeling you were focusing on has been released.

Client feels worse?

If the client reports feeling *worse*, check to see if the discomfort being experienced is the *same feeling*. For example, you may have started out releasing a feeling of frustration, and now the client reports feeling anger. Anger feels worse than frustration, but it's not the same feeling.

When the client reports feeling worse, bring attention back to the feeling you were releasing on and say, "A moment ago, you were feeling frustrated. Are you still feeling frustrated or is it something else?"

If the client confirms that the original (frustrated) feeling is gone, validate the change that has just occurred. They have successfully released an uncomfortable feeling! Change is occurring! What they're doing is working! Get the client on a roll by validating each increment of change. For example, "I let something go! If I can feel it, I can heal it! I'm allowed to release everything unlike love and feel better. I look forward to more of this!" This establishes a new level of trust while setting up for the next wave of emotional releasing.

> *Validation in the pharmaceutical and medical device industry is defined as the documented act of demonstrating that a procedure, process, and activity will consistently lead to the expected results.* ~ **Online Dictionary**

If the client reports that the feeling of frustration has changed to anger, ask, "What happened to the frustration?" Validate that change has occurred. Then, point out that a deeper level is surfacing. That's good! Offer the suggestion, "Love brings up everything unlike itself to be healed.[29]" Then, reassure your client that you will take care of that feeling in a moment, but first, you want to make sure that the frustrated feeling is completely gone.

Remember, that feeling is like infection in an open wound. Healing requires a complete releasing of the feeling. Before proceeding, check to make sure "that feeling" has been neutralized. Invite the client to go inside and try to find the frustrated feeling. Is it *all* gone?

If the client reports that that feeling is *the same*, this could indicate that you're right on target. It's just that there's a lot more "volume" present than the client was initially aware of. This is what they have been avoiding! Be persistent. It can take many rounds to get it all out.

---

[29] Sondra Ray

Find out if the intensity has changed. Perhaps something *was* let go but there's still something left. Take a Subjective Unit of Distress (SUD). Normally, you take a SUD level to establish a baseline before beginning the releasing process, but you can also take a SUD retroactively. Ask the client, "How strong was that (frustrated) feeling to begin with? On a scale of one to ten, where ten is the worst that it has ever been, how strong was that feeling?" Then, ask the client to rate that feeling *now*.

If the feeling has come down *at all*, validate the change! Do a little math to point out the percentage of change that has occurred. For example: If it started out as a ten and it's now a five, that's a 50% improvement. That's something worth celebrating, isn't it? Validate it! "I feel better! A moment ago, I was feeling really uncomfortable! But I *do* feel better. I let something go! I look forward to more of this! Even though there's still *some* of that frustrated feeling still there, I'm allowed to feel it, and I'm allowed to release it to feel better!" This helps the client recognize how much better she *does* feel. It also provides evidence that change is occurring.

Help the client to recognize that healing is a process, and the process is working. Then, set up for the next round of releasing by asking, "Do you want to keep that remaining (five) or release it?" With the client's permission, bring attention back to the *remaining* frustration, in this case the remaining five, and continue releasing until it's down to a zero. Once the feeling is completely neutralized, you can move onto releasing the next feeling (in this case, anger).

If the feeling doesn't seem to be releasing, get more specific by adding a "because" statement. For example, "I still feel frustrated because (put an ending on it)". Or "the thought of X still makes me feel frustrated *because* (put an ending on it)."

If the client says, "I still feel frustrated because …" but offers a new reason (thought), he could be experiencing another aspect or "flavor" of frustration. Give the suggestion that a deeper layer is coming to the surface and praise the client's good work! The next step is then to release on the new thought/feeling/perception until the client reports a shift to the better. Then, validate that change!

When the SUD is down to a zero ask the client to tell you what, specifically, has changed. For example, "What's changed? How do you know it's changed?" As the client describes what's different *now*, they are reinforcing the perception that *they* are changing for the better. You can then continue with a mini review. For example: "For example, "I feel better. A moment ago, I felt angry in my (gut). But *now* I feel … (put an ending on it.)" Often the client will say, with surprise, "Calm!" or "Relaxed." That's an insight! The client is realizing change is happening. Grab it! Grab every opportunity to celebrate positive change. This will open the door to allow more change to happen.

Moments of insight and recognition of change offer you the opportunity to formulate potent suggestions based on the client's own truth. For example: "I *do* feel better! I feel calm! I can feel it in my body! This is my feeling! I'm allowed to feel better! A moment ago, I was feeling (scared). And now I feel calm! I'm allowed to feel calm, like I do right now. I look forward to more of this feeling!"

The key is to reinforce every success, no matter how small. As you guide your clients through the process, watch for visible signs of release. Sighing, yawning, shifts in vocal tone, appearing calmer, sounding more self-assured, mature, etc. are signs that the body is relaxing and that the feeling is losing its hold.

Bring the client's attention to these small shifts. Help them to realize that change is happening! If you sense that the client may have already released the feeling, you can test by asking, "It's changing, isn't it?"

If the client confirms that the feeling has, indeed shifted, shift to using past tense, "The thought of X *made* me feel (angry) …. and it's changing." For example:

Eyebrow = "The thought of X makes me feel angry!"

Side of Eye = "The thought of X makes me feel angry!"

Under Eye = "Feeling angry with the thought of X."

Under Nose = "This anger with the thought of X."

Collar Bone = "The thought of X makes me feel angry" (client takes a deep breath and relaxes)

→ *"It's changing, isn't it?"* (Client nods)

Heart = "The thought of X *made me feel angry … and it's changing* "(validating the change)

Top of Head = "The thought of X made me feel angry … and it's changing"

Index Finger = "The thought of X made me feel angry … and it's changing"

Middle Finger = "The thought of X made me feel angry … and *I'm* changing" (integrating the change)

Little Finger = "And even though the thought of X made me feel angry … I'm changing"

Karate Chop = "I'm changing … because I accept my feelings… even the angry ones … And I deeply and completely accept myself."

Once you have released all the aspects contributing to the problem, test the results by asking the client to do a review of the situation/event. When the client can tell the whole story without being triggered, it's a done deal.

If it's totally clear, validate this new level of awareness. Then, seal the deal with direct suggestions to reinforce whatever positive changes have *already* occurred.

Notice how this is different than just reading a script? Instead of trying to suggest that something is true (when it isn't), you focus on identifying and releasing the internal objections that prevent the client from accepting more positive suggestions for change. When all the aspects contributing to the problem have been released and resolved, suggestions for change will be readily accepted. This is why you must test to ensure that the release is complete. You are not offering suggestions to make a change. You are suggesting what is already true for the client. This encourages a deeper level of integration of that truth.

Releasing the blocks will result in an internal shift. Validating each shift will allow for another shift, and then another . . . Once the subconscious mind catches on, a generalizing effect will occur to bring these changes into alignment with a new way of being for the client. In this way, you can incrementally walk the client right out of the problem.

Feelings don't come out of nowhere. The underlying cause of the problem has to do with decisions that are being made during an emotionally charged life experience. This is what Stephen Parkhill called Thought-Cause Alignment. This is what you're looking for during the uncovering procedure.

~ **The Devil's Therapy**: *Hypnosis Practitioner's Essential Guide to Effective Regression Hypnotherapy*

CHAPTER 10: INNER CHILD?

Inner Child Work is central to the work of regression hypnotherapy because Child Parts are feeling Parts. They are shaped by events very early in life and form our Core Beliefs. Each Part has its own memories and individual point of view, based on past experiences and what was learned from them. As such, it can be a source of empowerment or a problem depending on how it's expressing in a person's life." – **The Devil's Therapy**

Inner Child Work is Parts Therapy. In regression hypnotherapy, the goal is to facilitate the Inner Child Work within the event that caused the Part to form. This is the event that is responsible for generating symptoms and/or unwanted behavior(s). Parts can form at any age but the ones that form before the formation of the Critical Faculty of the mind are responsible for core beliefs which shape identity.

There isn't just one Inner Child. There are many, many Inner Child Parts - one for every event. The problem is that some of these Parts are in distress because they're stuck in the traumatic event that caused them to form in the first place. This keeps the client stuck in the pain story. The pain story is a narrative constructed by the client at a younger age. This story is based on experiences, both real and imagined, and is informed by the perceptions, thoughts, and feelings of the Child.

You cannot erase, delete, banish, or amputate a Part of the client. If you try, you will do damage. Every Part serves an important purpose. Child Parts are feeling parts. Fear serves a positive purpose. Anger serves a positive purpose. Sadness serves a positive purpose. The goal of Inner Child Work is not to get rid of the problematic part. Rather, it is to love the Part back to its natural state of wholeness.

Depression is a suppression of feeling. It, too, serves a positive purpose, but keeping a lid on your feelings can develop into physical symptoms later in life. This is because feelings buried alive don't die. They continue to strive for recognition. This is called the Symptom Imperative.

Any attempt to get rid of a symptom will make the problem worse by driving it underground where it will continue to fester. While merely treating the symptoms may yield temporary relief, sooner or later, the underlying problem will find its way to the surface through a recurrence of symptoms, recidivism, or conversion. [30]

The goal of Inner Child Work is not to change what happened in a past event. It's to change how the event was interpreted by the Inner Child and, therefore, how it feels. If something really happened, you can't change that, nor should you try. Any attempt to alter the truth, as the subconscious mind has it, would establish a false memory. No matter how well-intentioned, implanting false memories can only make matters worse by generating internal conflict.

---

[30] The Devil's Therapy: Hypnosis Practitioner's Essential Guide to Effective Regression Hypnotherapy

You can't lie to the subconscious mind. It knows the truth. It's just that the subconscious truth is not necessarily based on facts. It's based on the perceptions of the Child and the age and maturity of the Child at the time the event occurred.

Perceptions are how the Child experiences five-sensory input from its environment. Whatever the Child is seeing, hearing, smelling, tasting, and touching in that situation is being evaluated and interpreted as either "good" or "bad." Sweet is good, sour is yucky. Being cuddled is good, being molested is bad. Meaning is then assigned to this experience. Based on this meaning, decisions are then made. For example, an experience of abuse may generate the thought, "I'm going to die!" This thought then gets anchored to specific triggers associated with the causal event. The trigger could be anything - a certain sound, color, the look on someone's face, a particular tone of voice, a smell, a physical gesture or even a random object or color.

In future, every time the Child encounters the same trigger – seeing, hearing, smelling, tasting, or touching – that stimulus will act as a reminder of the "first time", triggering a cascade of thoughts, feelings and responses formed during the ISE. The Child doesn't even have to experience something directly. A child witnessing an act of violence will perceive it as a personal threat. This is due to mirror neurons which help us to learn through observation. But the emotions generated by witnessing violence will register as a traumatic experience, generating feelings of physical tension which will feel uncomfortable. The child will then try to make sense of what's happening. Whatever meaning is given to the situation will form the basis of decisions about self, others, and life. For example, a young child might decide, "It's my fault" or "I did something to cause this." Children often take the blame when bad things happen in their world.

Our earliest decisions form the basis of core beliefs. Core beliefs tell us how to be and not-be to survive. They shape identity and our ability to trust ourselves and others. They tell us what to expect from ourselves and others, and how relationships should work. They tell us whether the world is a safe place and when we should run for cover. The problem is that decisions that are made early in life are based on the cognitive and emotional maturity of a child. Remember, prior to age five or six, a child lacks the ability to discriminate between real and imagined, true or false.

Inner Child Work can be done in any event, but the goal is to thoroughly process the ISE because that's the seed-planting event for the problematic pattern.

The Steps:

1. Uncover the story.
2. Prepare the Grownup.
3. Prepare the child.
4. Find the thought-feeling.
5. Reality-check the thought
6. Find the good.
7. Grow the Child up.

Step 1: Uncover the story.

Guide the client to step into the event, then conduct the preliminary uncovering process to get a general sense of what happened, where it happened, and who was involved in the event. What's the story?

If the client is apprehensive about stepping into the event, you can help to reduce resistance by reminding them that this is only a memory, and that there's nothing here that they haven't already lived through. It's just that the subconscious mind doesn't know this, yet. "We're here to change that so you can feel better."

Step 2: Prepare the Grownup.
Once the initial uncovering work is complete, guide the client back to *before* the event plays out. Nothing "bad" has happened yet, so before the event, the Child will be feeling good. Place the Child in the background so you can have a talk with the client. Then, prepare the client to be a loving support for their Inner Child.

The client's job is to take on the role of the good parent for their Inner Child. This begins with expressing love and acceptance for the Child, then promising to be there for the Child from now on. This provides the Child with something that was missing during the original experience – a source of security. Bringing in adult consciousness to educate and support the Child solves the most fundamental problem of any ISE which was having to deal with a distressing situation *alone*. The client then prepares the Child for what is *about to happen* in the ISE.

Step 3: Prepare the Child.
The ISE always begins with an initial shock to the nervous system. The Child didn't see it coming. It was totally new and unexpected. As a result, it put the Child into a stress response. But a huge part of the distress has to do with not-knowing. The Child cannot predict what's going to happen next. This naturally results in fear and anxiety. Informing the Child about what is *about* to happen changes that and can reduce a significant amount of resistance.

What the Child most needs to know is:
- She will get through the event; she will survive,

- She doesn't have to face it alone; Grownup will be with her every step of the way,
- She gets to grow up; Grownup is living proof of this.

Once the Child has been informed about what's going to happen, the event plays out exactly as it did the first time. The only thing that has changed is that the Child now knows what she didn't know the first time - that she will survive and grow up to adulthood. Adult consciousness is then present to provide what the Child most needed - love and support in making sense of the experience.

Step 4: Find the thought-feeling.

Herein lies the key to transforming a traumatic experience in childhood. It's in uncovering how the Child was making sense of what was happening.

- What's happening?
- What does that make you think?
- How does that make you feel?

What are the unmet needs of the Child in that event? How can Grownup meet those needs now that they're known?

Step 5: Reality-check the thought.

The thought is the cause of the feeling. You need to reality check the thought with Grownup. Is it true? If it's not true, re-educate the Child about what *is* true. For example, the Child thinks that Mom is abandoning her. She thinks Mom is never going to come back. That's generating fear. But the truth is, Mom is dropping the Child off at daycare for the first time, and Mom's only going to be gone for a few hours. The Child can now feel safe and realize there are other children to play with.

If the Child's interpretation of the situation is not accurate, invite Grownup to tell the Child the truth about what's happening. Ask, "What does the Child most need to know to get through the event feeling okay?" or "If you'd known then, what you know now, how might that have changed things?" Providing the Child with this information removes the initial shock of the ISE.

If it's true, the next step is to help the client come to acceptance. It happened. You can't just rewrite a memory. You must transform the memory by changing how it *feels*.

The way to transform how a memory feels is to help the Child get through the event without being negatively impacted by it. Release the emotional charge then reframe what happened.

If the Child's interpretation of what's happening is true, what's needed is acceptance and forgiveness. In this case, validate the perceptions and feelings of the Child. Then, find a way to bring the client to a place of recognition. It happened. It's sad but true. And while it wasn't the greatest experience, *it's over*. Help the client to realize that the past is the past. This allows the subconscious mind to finally relax. That's when healing happens.

Step 6: Find the good
It's a foul wind that doesn't blow any good, and every cloud has a silver lining. What could the Child learn from this experience that would serve her in future? What's the nugget of wisdom, the gift in the garbage? How might realizing this change things in future?

Step 7: Grow the Child up.

Transforming the narrative about what happened in the ISE, how it affected the client, and how it developed into a life story changes the client's experience of growing up the SSEs.

The ISE doesn't change. The SSEs will automatically change because the client has changed as result of resolving the ISE. Because the Child is no longer stuck in the erroneous perceptions, thoughts and feelings at the ISE, everything about the client is undergoing change.

As you grow the client up through the SSEs, they are rewriting history. This is the client's life story. It has power. It defines them. It decides what they can expect in the future because of their past experiences. It is creating their reality NOW. By changing the beginning of the story (ISE), the client's overall lens on life changes. As a result, everything changes for the better.

Help the client to realize that change is occurring as you guide her forward in time. She's growing and changing because she's no longer stuck in the past. Validate every insight and recognition of change.

Troubleshooting the Inner Child Work

Adult does not feel love for Child?

When Grownup cannot feel love toward their inner child, do not proceed with the Inner Child Work. It's not that they can't feel love or that they've never experienced love. It's that they have become disconnected from their true self. It's because events in life, growing up, have conditioned them into a negative bias. This is common with depression.

No matter how awful their childhood might have been, they survived it. Research from wartime orphanages shows that children who are deprived of love don't survive. They give up and die. This tells you that there must have been some love. The problem is that the client is unable to find it because of the heavy blanket of negative expectations. That's the block.

The block is what the client is paying you to resolve. Release it and they'll start feeling better, almost immediately. You just need to take things slow and easy. If you try to force your way past a subconscious block, you're going to increase resistance and, with it, the negativity.

Remember, the subconscious mind's Prime Directive is to protect. That block is there for a reason. The harder you push, the more pushback you're going to get. BUT . . . if you use a gentle, patient approach, you can coax the subconscious mind into cooperating. Why? Because you are demonstrating a loving approach. You are showing that you care enough not to bully the client into submission. You're not pushing your agenda on the client. You're demonstrating that you accept them where they're at. That's love. And love heals.

Deep within you is the wisdom to know how to guide the client into a better place. But to do this, you need to recognize that you are dealing with a very wounded Child. The walls are there to protect a vulnerable, frightened, hurting little one whose needs have gone unmet for far too long. Your ability to demonstrate loving care and attention can make it safe enough for that wounded little one to come out. Take your time. Build resources. Deal with the layers of grief which include fear, anger, and guilt.

I would use a Stems Completion Exercise with a focus on positive aspects. Invite the client to tell you something they love. "Something I love is . . . (put an ending on it)" Think raindrops on roses and whiskers on kittens. For example, did the client ever have a special pet? Did they love that pet? How do they know that? Where do they feel "that feeling"? Did they have a grandparent or a teacher who cared about them?

If you can access a better feeling, you can anchor it in. You then have a starting point from which to grind down to a better feeling. Find a positive feeling. Locate it in the body. Increase attention on "that feeling" to amplify the feeling. Allow the feeling to be there. Then, find another feeling. Keep grinding down until you find the love.

Another approach you can use is the hypermnesia exercise. You don't need hypnosis for this but, if you induce somnambulism first, you can very quickly convert it to a real regression. When a person is very strongly biased to the negative, positive memories can elicit negative emotions. If you're dealing with a deeply depressed client, trying to push them into a positive feeling will cause them to spiral down into a deep hole.

Child feels 'anxious'?

Anxiety can be anticipatory fear or dread. Because it's referencing a past event, you're not dealing with a new feeling which means that you haven't yet located the ISE. The problem with "anxiety" is that it's a very grownup word for a common childhood problem. Find the Child's word for "that feeling" and you'll access a more authentic feeling for Affect Bridge. For example, "That anxious feeling in your gut . . . what emotion might it be? Scared? Sad? Mad? Glad? Or something else?"

Child feels worthless?

When the Child reports feeling "not good enough" or "worthless", (both thoughts) keep the focus on the feeling in the body and grind down to the emotion. For example, "The thought 'not good enough' makes me feel (put an ending on it.)" Or, "The thought 'I'm worthless' makes me feel (put an ending on it.)" What emotion might that feeling be?

Whose expectations is the Child trying to live up to? Who are they trying to please? Reality Check it with Grownup. Are these expectations realistic?

Child doesn't 'feel right'?

Ask, "What is it about what's happening that doesn't feel *loving* to you?"

Child feels 'sad'?

Make sure the emotion is congruent with what's happening in the event. Sadness can be a mask for other emotions. For example, women are often socialized to cry when they feel angry or frustrated.

Authentic sadness has to do with a loss. If sadness is congruent with the situation ask, "What did you lose?" Let the Child tell you. Then, give permission to feel it fully.

Unresolved grief is painful. Use a maternal tone and guide the client to release the feeling by saying, "You let yourself be as hurt by that as you need to be. You get the cry out you'll feel so good."

If the feeling of sadness doesn't seem to be congruent with what's happening in the event, bring attention to the feeling in the body, then grind down to the real emotion.

Child feels 'lost'?

If the client reports feeling lost or says, "I lost myself," that's the voice of depression. Depression is *suppression* of a true emotion. Often, what's behind it is anger.

Child feels 'depressed'?

If the client is feeling depressed, you're not in the ISE. Depression is a last-ditch effort at pain-relief by putting a lid on the emotion. Regress back to the point where "it just wasn't worth it to feel that feeling, anymore."

Child feels 'confused'?

Confusion is the inability to make sense of what's happening in your environment. What's needed is understanding. Say, "Your mind rewinds, and the whole scene plays out, again. This time, your mind is able to put it all together. Everything you've learned in the session, so far, comes together in an understanding."

Young children compartmentalize their feelings. They lack the emotional maturity needed to experience competing feelings. If the client is experiencing mixed emotions, identify the strongest emotion and follow it back. The stronger the feeling, the more staying power it will have when you're Bridging back.

If confusion follows an initial shock/surprise in the event, you may have found the ISE.

Child feels 'nothing'?

This is a block to allowing the feeling. The only people who feel 'nothing' are dead. By-pass the block by Bridging back to the event where the Child decided to shut down her feelings. For example, "Sometimes, nothing is something. Focus on that 'nothing' feeling. As

I count from three down to one, your mind takes us to an event that has everything to do with it not being worth feeling your feelings."

Client is 'crying'?

When tears find their way to the surface, bring the client's attention to them. Encourage the client to let "that cry" out.

Match the client's emotional energy with your tonality. If the client is sobbing gently, use a very maternal voice and gently dab their cheek with a tissue while pouring in soothing suggestions. For example, "That's right. You just let yourself feel it all. We want every last ounce of that cry out of you. You're going to feel soooo goooood."

If the client is wailing in despair, raise the timbre of your voice and encourage them to get it all out. For example, "All the hurt. All the pain. All the sadness. Get. It. Out. You get that out, you're going to feel so good!"

Do *not* offer them a tissue. This will distract their attention away from feeling the feeling and can even shut down the feeling. If the client is generating a lot of snot, and begins gagging or choking, place a wad of tissues in their lap to give them something to spit into. But keep them focused on the feeling and encourage the client to feel it fully.

If the client tries to wipe away their tears, they're likely feeling self-conscious. This brings in the conscious mind. Stop them! Keep them focused on the truth of "that feeling." For example, "Don't wipe it away. Let it be as messy as it needs to be. You've spent your whole life wiping it away. There's only one place that can hurt you, and that's trapped inside. You get that out and it no longer has any control over your life."

Child feels 'hurt'?

Hurt can mean sadness and/or anger. It can point to betrayal, disappointment, abandonment, rejection, and loss. Validate the client's right to take the lid off that feeling and let it express. For example, "You let yourself be as hurt by that as you need to be. Everybody else is trying to teach you to hold this in, to be a tough little soldier, suck in your gut. This is probably the first time somebody tells you it's okay to feel your feelings. It's okay to get it all out. All the pain and tears and sadness. Let it all out. You're allowed to be as disturbed, and hurt, and sad by that information as you need to be. Find the words and get it out, you'll feel so good. No more tough little soldier, no more holding it in, no more trying to figure it all out, understand? (Snap, snap, snap) Every word that ever got swallowed away."

Child feels 'anger, hate, frustration'?

Peeved, pissed, frustrated, furious, hate, etc. describe degrees of anger. The antidote for anger is forgiveness. The way to get forgiveness is through the process of releasing the anger. This is the purpose of Pillow Therapy. Your pillow provides a big target for bigger emotions like anger.

Instruct the client to find the words that need to be said and to *pump* the feeling into the pillow. For example, "At the count of three, (tap client's arm) your arm becomes an extension of your subconscious mind. All the emotions come down into your arm. Your subconscious mind speaks through your arm. You get it all out. You don't want an ounce of it to remain. GET IT OUT! Get it *all* out. All that (frustration) trapped inside for all those years comes out. Everything (he's) ever done - get it out until it's all gone. One, two, three! Find the words. You'll know when there's nothing left."

Client feels 'guilt or shame'?

Guilt and shame are thoughts. Really, they're just two sides of the same coin. Guilt is the thought that says, "I *did* something wrong/bad." This thought generates the fear of punishment. Children often take the blame for the things that happen to them. As a result, this separates them from themselves. You can repair this during the forgiveness process by separating the internalized representation of the Offender from the client. Then, release the anger toward the Offender to remove the self-punishment program.

When the client reports guilt, reality-check the Child's assessment of the situation with adult consciousness. For example, "Grownup, (Child) thinks that he's done something wrong. Is that true?"

If the Child did something 'wrong', what's needed is acceptance and encouragement in learning an important lesson. Human beings learn through trial and error. What is the Child learning that can help her in future?

Shame is the root cause of every addiction. Shame is a barrage of thoughts that say, "There is something wrong with me. I'm bad, I'm defective, broken, flawed, beyond redemption (and therefore, unlovable, worthless and beyond hope)." This generates grief and profound despair.

When the client reports shame, take them back to before they knew what it was like to feel "that shame". Find their innocent Inner Child and help the client to reclaim this Part of herself.

Remember, the adult consciousness of the client is the accumulated pain of a lifetime. The Child is the gold! Take the client back to recognize the Truth so they can heal. Say, "As I count from three down to one, your mind takes us back to an earlier time, where all the Child knew was love. Go all the way back to that moment when all she knew was how loveable she was."

You may have to go back into the womb, but when you find that moment of pure innocence, saturate the client's mind and body with that feeling of love. Then, send it forward along their timeline. For example, "Send that love, and all the good feelings, forward now, transforming every moment in your life, and every experience that, in any way, conflicts with the truth about you. Because the truth about you is . . . *you are you.* And that's enough. You're *good* enough. You're *lovable* enough. You're *worthy* enough. (Add suggestions to correct any perceived inadequacy reported by the Child such as "smart enough" or "creative enough".)

"You are enough . . . *not because I say so* but because you always have been. There's nothing wrong with you. There never was. It's just that sometimes we forget. We all do it. But the truth is . . . (if the client is spiritual, "you have a Creator, and your Creator knows that) . . . You were *made* always loveable. From now on, you get to know that and feel that way, too. Always remember that. You are loved. Because . . . *this time* . . . you get to grow up always *remembering* the truth about you. You are you . . . a worthy soul on an important journey, always loveable, etc.

"On the count of three, begin moving forward along your timeline. One, two, three . . . moving forward now, through the childhood years into adolescence . . . knowing only the love. Further now, through the teens and into early adulthood, etc." (Continue right up to the adult in the here and now, sitting in your chair. Integrate the changes. Repeat the process to compound the changes.)

Child thinks "I'm not wanted"?

A common decision in childhood is "I'm not wanted." Sometimes it's true. Often, it's a misinterpretation of the situation. Either way, regression hypnotherapy does not gloss over the truth of how it was for the client in childhood. Validate the feelings of the Child, then test for the ISE. For example, "These things that you're discovering (this feeling that she doesn't want you) . . . is this a surprise . . . or knowledge you have? What's your first sense?" (i.e., "new or familiar".)

If being "not wanted" is familiar to the Child, locate the earlier event where this knowledge comes as a surprise. Then, reality-check the perceptions of the Child in the ISE by asking adult consciousness, "Is that true?"

If the Child's perception of not being-wanted is *not* true, simply have Grownup inform the Child of the truth to correct the problem.

If the Child's perception is true, the goal becomes bringing the client to acceptance so that the Child can be informed of the truth and grow up feeling good about herself.

First, shift the responsibility onto the Offender. For example, if it's true that Mom doesn't want the Child, it's not the Child's fault. Establish a basis of truth by suggesting, "Mom has the problem, the Child's not the problem, isn't that true?"

Then, validate the Child's truth. "(Child) thinks there's something wrong with her. She doesn't know that Mom's got the problem. (Child's) not the problem. All (Child) wants or needs is to be loved and accepted, isn't that true?"

You can then use more general suggestion regarding what *every* Child needs, for example, "to feel safe and secure, to know that she is loved and accepted, and to grow up knowing the truth about here - that there is nothing wrong with her."

Once you have established the truth about the Child, you can begin the reparenting process where the Grownup client assumes the role of loving and protective guide to the Inner Child.

Client can't find any good?
If the client is struggling to find some good in a "bad situation", they're holding onto blame. Remember, that blame has been turned inward. This keeps the client stuck in Victim Stance. Finding the good for *the Child* allows the Child to grow up bringing more resources into adulthood. For example, "We're not making excuses here, but only recognizing that every cloud has a silver lining, understand?"

Traumatic experiences early in life impact identity. Finding the good reverses the harmful effects by reframing the event as resilience training. The fact is, she survived! That took courage! How might this have made her stronger? What did she learn from that situation? What did she learn about self/others? How might this knowledge empower her in the future? How might she use this knowledge to help/empower others? For example, leadership skills, friendship skills, etc.

How might that experience have made her more resourceful? For example, what unique skills or knowledge might she have gained through this experience? What values, purpose, sense of identity can be identified and claimed?

If something was done to her, would she ever do that to someone she cared about? Would she protect those she loves from something similar? If so, "So, it made you wiser, huh?"

Childhood abuse?

Childhood abuse is seldom a one-time event. Repetition, over time, ensures that the pattern will be reinforced, making it stronger. Eventually, the unresolved pain story will find expression through symptoms. This is how phobias are formed.

If the client bumps into a repetitive traumatic event pattern, you don't have to process every single event of abuse. You can condense the event *pattern* into a single event and release it *as if* it were a single event. For example, "Every time (event pattern) has happened gets condensed into one event, and you get it all out."

Once the purging process is complete, review the event to test for residual aspects. For example, "I know this event really seems bad to the mind but watch what happens. On the count of one, that 'one big event' rewinds and replays, only this time it's not as bad as it seems. After all, you already lived through it once (pause). Maybe there's nothing there. All the emotions leave. What matters here is that you don't hide from your feelings. You get it out. You (cry it out, pump it out, choke it out, etc.) Whatever it takes, you get it out until there's nothing left. Then you're free of it. Understand?"

No Time to Find the ISE?

When a client bounces back into a painful event in the first session, you might not have enough time to process the whole event. In this case, you need to button up your session in readiness for the next session. Buttoning up allows you to come back to where you left off and finish up the work in the next session.

If you don't have enough time in your session to get to the ISE, no worries. Being client-centered means the client decides the time it takes. All you need to do is find a way to give the client some relief and use it to instill confidence in the process. To button up your session, validate the better feeling and then reframe the event.

Validate the feeling. When you validate a feeling, you are giving value to the Subconscious Mind and what it has to say. "That feeling" is an important Part of the client. It has been brought to awareness for a reason.

Every feeling is a worthy Part of the client. It deserves to be loved, accepted, and forgiven. Give it permission to be there by helping the client to recognize that their subconscious mind is not the enemy. Their emotions are not 'bad' or 'wrong.' The problem they've been struggling with has everything to do with past events.

Reframe the event. Once you have validated the client's right to feel all their feelings, find a way to turn their experience during the session into a revelation. What have they just discovered? What are they learning? Make these realizations into a breakthrough moment in the client's healing by tying them to the client's Therapeutic Goal. For example, how did that past experience contribute to the weight problem, or the skin problem, or the relationship problem?

Reinforce the benefits. Wrap your session up by reminding the client of the change they want and all the benefits of having made that change. Then, deliver the suggestion that *the process has already begun*. And that, as you continue to work together, more will be revealed to allow a complete healing of the problem.

Not sure you found the ISE?

You can process any SSE *as if* it were the ISE. Then, button things up in a way that allows you to come back to where you left off in the next session. Next session, complete the process of locating the ISE.

If you're not certain that you've located the ISE, but you're running out of time, process the event *as if* it were the ISE. If the SSE is close to the ISE, it can have a backwash effect into the ISE, weakening it or even dissolving it. Bring in adult consciousness and teach the client how to support and love their Inner Child. Then, give the suggestion to ripple those changes forward and backward along the timeline. Finally, grow the Child up to adulthood.

Next session, go back to this event and see if you can bring up the emotion. If there's even a whisper of emotion still trapped in the event, amplify "that feeling", then Bridge back to the "first time" they ever felt that feeling.

No time to complete Inner Child Work?

If you have located the ISE but don't have time to completely resolve it, the Child is still in distress. You can provide much-needed safety for the Child by placing the Child in the client's heart. This places the responsibility for the care and keeping of this important Part in the hands of the client. For example, before emerging the client, invite them to generate feelings of love and acceptance for their Inner Child. Send those energies into the Child. Then, find a place in the heart where the Child can go and always know that she is safe and loved.

Once you have placed the Child in that safe place inside of the client, invite the client to notice how it feels. What's that like? How does the Child like being in there? Does she feel safe and secure?

If the Child is feeling safe and secure inside the heart, remind the client that they have something precious inside of them. Then, instruct the client to only say nice things to herself because the "little one" is listening. You can then say, "Put a bookmark on that event so that we can come back to it, later." This is a post-hypnotic suggestion to return to the same event in a future session establishing a starting point for the next session.

Next session, do a brief review during the pre-hypnosis interview to stir up the memory of that specific event. Then, use a directed regression to return to the event, do a quick review, and continue with the healing process.

No time to grow the Child up through the SSEs?
Wrap up the session with suggestions that tie the changes that have occurred in the event to the client's Therapeutic Goal and remind the client of the desired benefits. Make whatever happened in the session relevant to the client's desired outcome.

Next session, return to the event and pick up where you left off. Bring up the emotion, amplify it, and continue to release the thought and emotional energies trapped in the ISE.

Is the ISE clear?
When an event has been neutralized, the client will be able to review the experience as an observer. There will be no emotional charge, present. This is the time to elicit insights before progressing through the SSEs. What is the client learning? Ask, "What's changed?" Validate those changes. Then ask, "How might this change things in the future?"

As you progress through the SSEs, test and compound all changes. When you reach the level of adult awareness, integrate the accumulation of changes – physically, mentally, and emotionally. Then, Future Pace to test the client's expectations for the future.

If the future looks bright, bring this newer, better level of awareness back into the client's here and now as a *vision for the future* that she is now living into.

No time to clear the ISE?

If you don't have enough time to thoroughly clear everything in the ISE, button it up in a way that allows you to pick up where you left off in the next session.

1. Place the Child in the client's heart. "That way, she'll always feel safe. And you'll always know that you have something precious inside of you."
2. Give the suggestion, "Put a bookmark on this event so we can come back to it, later."
3. Fade the scene and return attention to feeling of the back pressing down into the chair. Then say, "Well, now we know."
4. Tie the experience to the client's therapeutic goal. For example, "That situation/event has everything to do with (presenting problem)."
5. Acknowledge the courage it took for the client to face their feeling/past.
6. Build enthusiasm for continuing the work. For example, "You can look forward to resolving (presenting problem) for good!"
7. Remind the client of any insights or better feelings resulting from the process. Use them as validations that the healing process is working.

8. Validate every step in the right direction. Praise every accomplishment, no matter how small.
9. Emerge the client with gusto!

During the post-hypnosis debrief, ask the client, "What did you discovered as a result of the process?" This will help to reinforce learning at a conscious level. Validate the client's willingness to let herself feel her feelings. Remind her that holding onto the feeling is the problem and has been costing her their quality of life.

Finally:

- Schedule the next session within one week.
- Remind the client to pay attention to her feelings between sessions so that she can report back to you anything of significance in the next session.
- Next session, do a directed regression to the event, repeat the uncovering procedure to bring up the feeling, and continue on.

No Time for Future Pacing?

Wrap up your session with suggestions to reinforce all changes. Then, send the client off to test the results between sessions. Next session, if the client has been able to hold onto the changes, give them a yummy relaxation hypnosis session with heaps of compounding suggestions.

Begin with a review of the journey you've taken the client on. Use the client's own insights to tell them the Child's story of learning, and growing, and becoming more (fill in the blank with qualities the client has reclaimed through the process.) For example, more calm, confident, safe, worthy, proud, in control, etc. Then, generalize all changes "throughout all time and space" by gathering up all the positive changes and sending them back to the moment of conception. Drop the changes into the client's timeline and have them ripple forward through all the SSEs into the client's here and now.

As this happens, give suggestions that amplify all the benefits. For example, "growing and expanding" the better thoughts and feeling. Then, invite the client to embody these changes at the adult level of awareness – physically, mentally, emotionally, spiritually - before sending them forward into the future.

If you have time, take the client forward in time to meet their Future Self. Guide them to have a conversation, then receive a gift or a promise from their older, wiser self. Bring what they gain back into the present time.

Be creative! Have fun!

The way out is always through.

– **Robert Frost**

CHAPTER 11:
TESTED & INTEGRATED?

No *matter how thorough you might be in addressing all the contributing aspects, there is no guarantee that you have found all the roots of the client's problem. Deeper layers of truth can be withheld until the subconscious mind feels that it's safe to reveal them. So, you won't necessarily uncover the whole Story right away. The client can consciously choose to withhold some piece of information because they judge it unimportant or too shameful to admit to. But if it's not brought to light, you can't fix it. Whatever the client fails to disclose is still there, calling for release. Left unresolved, the problem will persist. This is why you must test the results.* – **The Devil's Therapy**

Once the Inner Child Work is complete, the next step is to grow the Child up through the SSEs. Growing the Child up through the SSEs gives you a way to integrate all changes and:

1. Test to make sure the ISE is clear.
2. Take care of dust-bunnies.
3. Clear secondary aspects.

Test to make sure the ISE is clear.

Growing the Child up through the SSEs allows you to encourage further integration of all changes while testing for any unresolved aspects that may still be trapped in the ISE.

When growing the Child up, if you bump into a block in an SSE, stop right there and identify whether this is a new aspect or an unresolved hangover from the ISE. If you find an emotion that was in the ISE, go back to the ISE and conduct the ISE test for "that feeling". There may be an earlier event or a secondary ISE feeding into the problem. Most of the time, it's something you missed in the ISE. In this case, go back and clear what's left in the ISE. Then, before progressing through the SSEs, again, test to make sure that the ISE is really and truly clear.

If the client bumps into a new feeling in an SSE, this is probably something that got added onto the symptom pattern after the ISE occurred. In this case, take a SUD. How strong is "that feeling." If it's a strong emotion (7 or higher), Bridge back to the ISE for "that feeling" and clear it in the causal event.

If it's a weak emotion, release it in the SSE. For example, if the SUD is a three, you can release it in the SSE. Then, run the event, again, to test to make sure it's gone. As you continue to progress through the SSEs, this change will be added to the changes being generalized throughout the mind-body system.

Take care of dust-bunnies

Growing the Child up through the SSEs allow you to identify and clear any 'dust-bunnies.' Dust-bunnies are small stuff that was dealt with in the ISE but may have a different context in an SSE. These minor issues can usually be resolved easily by reality-checking perceptions and applying direct suggestions.

Clear secondary aspects.
As you grow the Child up through the SSEs, you may come across emotional stuff that got added to the pain package over time. I call this the Snowball Effect. Usually, this is small stuff, which can be cleared easily by inviting the Child to "remember back" to the ISE and recognize how they have matured since then.

If you bump into a big feeling, don't try to suggest it away. Bridge back off it. There could be a secondary ISE.

Framing Technique

The Framing Technique[31] is a way to capture the essence of a healing and test for residual aspects in a specific event from the past. It also allows you to identify the specific emotional frequency that was "missing" in the original event.

After clearing the event, ask the client to take a 'snapshot' of the scene. This suggests taking a broader view of the event, encapsulating it into a single image. Then, suggest that the client just let the Subconscious Mind put a frame around it in a color of its own choosing.

Research in the field of color psychology is being used in advertising, food packaging, art, style, and decorating. Much of this research shows that color evokes a common physiological response in humans. This is an automatic response that is below the level of conscious awareness. Subconsciously, color represents an emotional state. Colors can reflect both positive and negative emotions. For example, the color red can indicate fiery enthusiasm, aliveness, sexual urges, or anger.

---

[31] Brent Baum, Healing Dimensions

There are also personal meanings assigned to specific colors which are based on personal experience. For this reason, it's best not to assume what a color might mean. For example, if the color of the frame is red or black, this could indicate that something is still unresolved. In this case, have the client focus on the color and notice how it feels. Ask the client, "Is it a good feeling or a not-so-good feeling?" The feeling associated with that color will tell you whether the event is clear.

If the event is clear, the color chosen for a frame will indicate what quality of emotion was missing in the original event. That quality is now being restored to memory at a Subconscious level of Mind.

Feelings don't come out of nowhere. What that color means to the client has everything to do with her personal history. If the feeling associated with the color is negative, you can use it as an entry-point for regression by naming the emotion, amplifying it, and Bridging back to the causal event.

If the feeling associated with the color is positive, make it stronger! You can amplify the feeling by flowing the color through the nervous system of the body[32]. Instruct the client to flow it through every part of the body – muscles, nerves, fiber, tendons, bone - saturating every cell down to the atomic level. This feels really good so slather it on and compound all the benefits!

---

[32] The body actually emits light on a daily basis. This light is 1,000 times less intense than levels that can be seen with the naked eye, but some people are able to see this light as the aura. Biophotons are the smallest physical units of light, which are stored in, and used by all biological organisms – including your body. These units of light may very well be in control of virtually every biochemical reaction that occurs in the body – including the body's ability to heal.

If the client is dealing with a physical condition, it's always important to "touch the owie." Have the client flow this specific "quality of (color)" into the afflicted organ. Then, ask the client to scan the body to see if there's any place the color didn't go. If there is, you have just uncovered another block. Focus on *that*.

If the color goes into every part of the body, symbolically every part of the client has accepted this quality. Amplify that color until it radiates outward beyond the body, cocooning the client in this new healing frequency.

If you find that you don't have enough time to grow the Child up through the SSEs, after clearing the ISE, here's a shortcut. Wrap the transformed scene in a ball of white light. Then, place the ball of light next to the client's heart. This places the Child inside the heart where it's safe. You can then suggest that the Child grows up quickly, all the way up to Adult Consciousness, knowing only safety, love and acceptance, and the positive qualities associated with that specific color.

When you reach Adult Consciousness, merge all these changes that have occurred into a single ball of white light. This instructs the Subconscious Mind to integrate these changes. When you combine all colors of the rainbow, you get white light. Invite the client to identify the essence of this quality of change by finding a word or a phrase for this newer, better frequency. You can then have the client step into the ball of white light or have him place it next to his heart.

Flow this energy throughout the Mind-Body system of the Adult client. Then, have the client imagine this ball of light expanding outward, surrounding him completely, and creating a protective cocoon.

You can reinforce the protective function with suggestions. For example, "Now that you have forgiven, you're so much more aware. You realize that only what is loving is true. If someone were ever to say or do something that, in the past might have upset you, it bounces right off. From now on, energetically, you're like Teflon. You attract only good qualities into your life. etc."

Timeline Generalization Technique

Once the ISE has been resolved, and you have processed all the SSE's, the client's life Story is undergoing dramatic change. The subconscious mind is revising the client's storyline. Remember, the subconscious mind naturally generalizes all change. Timeline Generalization[33] is a technique you can use to encourage this natural process. You can use it at the end of a session, or as a separate session, to compound all changes and integrate them as part of the client's life story.

Guide the client back to the ISE and instruct the client's subconscious mind to review and reinforce all the positive changes that have occurred there. This review process also helps the client to consciously recognize that change is occurring. To facilitate this, instruct the client to gather up all the learnings, new perceptions, insights, healing, self-worth, strength, and wisdom gained through the healing process. Then, have him take all these changes back to the moment before conception. Suggest that the client may see, or sense, or feel, or just know that his timeline is there below him and stretching into the future.

Once the client is aware of the timeline, instruct him to drop down into his timeline, carrying all these resources with him. This means that all the positive resources gained through the process of clearing the ISE

---

[33] Connierae Andreas, Core Transformation, 1994

can be there for the Child before the moment of conception. As a result, all these positive qualities and resources can now be available to the client *right from the beginning*.

Test the client's expectations (belief) of the benefits of change by asking, "How might having these positive qualities and resources, right from the start, *change things*?" How might this change things in general? How might this change things with respect to the presenting issue? What else might be changed as a result?

Gather up all these additional insights and realizations, as well. Then, instruct the client to drop down into the timeline and begin moving forward, bringing this new, expanded level of understanding and empowerment into every situation and event as he moves forward along the timeline. Suggest that, as he moves forward through time, each event is now being colored and transformed by these newer/beneficial energies. Remind him that the changes that are occurring inside the client are in alignment with his desired goal.

This can be a very quick process which allows the client to experience a more expansive sense of change. For example, you can give the client a moment of silence to do this.

Alternately, you can stretch it out by using an amplifying count. Or you can suggest moving through childhood years, teenage years, adulthood (decades for older clients) all the way up to the client relaxing in the chair. As soon as these changes have flowed fully into the client in the chair in the present, invite the client to give you a report. What has changed? Then, repeat the process to compound this *new level* of change. Go back to the beginning and send these energies forward along the timeline. Think of it as ironing out the wrinkles in time!

Once the client has experienced the process, subsequent passes can happen very quickly. Just suggest that the client "swooshes" along the timeline all the way up to their adult self in the chair, going deeper.

To complete the process, send the energies forward into future situations and events, both anticipated and unexpected. You can send it forward incrementally - three months, six months, one year - each time pausing to review what life is like now that these changes are operating fully in the client's life. Or you can just swoosh it forward along the timeline like a warm wave.

If, at any point during the process, you bump into a block, or some resistance, you know what to do. Focus on that feeling!

Moment of Insight (MOI)

The Moment of Insight is a technique I learned while training in 5-PATH™[34] that is very useful in helping a client to recognize and validate positive change as it is occurring during a session. You can use this Sentence Stems Completion exercise anytime during a regression session to reinforce an insight, encourage a deeper integration of learning, or empower the Child as she grows up through the SSEs.

The Moment of Insight involves three statements.

1. I have changed.
2. I know I have changed because . . .
3. Now I feel . . .

---

[34] 5-PATH is an acronym for Five Phase Advanced Transformational Healing. Originally, it stood for Five Phase Abreactive Therapeutic Hypnosis.

The first statement acknowledges a perceived change. That's the thought. The second statement provides evidence to support this perception, making the thought reasonable and, therefore, believable. This satisfies the conscious mind's need to understand. The third statement reinforces the change which has occurred emotionally. This satisfies the subconscious mind's need (to feel good) based on the thought (belief) suggested by the first statement thus making it real. To realize something is to "make real."

"I have changed."
Instruct the Child to say, "I have changed." Then, check to make sure this statement feels true. Always test your results! Ask the Child, "Does that feel true?"

If the client indicates that the statement feels true, give the instruction to repeat the statement and notice how it feels. This can generate the realization that something profound has just happened. That's the Wow! Factor. When this happens, the mind opens wide to accept suggestions for change.

"I know I have changed because."
The second instruction is for the Child to say, "I *know* I have changed *because* now I know (put an ending on it)."

"Now I feel."
The third statement is, "So now I *feel* (put an ending on it)." This is the real change. Regression Hypnotherapy doesn't change what happened. What changes is now the client feels about what happened by changing how it is being interpreted. That's the causal thought.

1. Thought. "I have changed."
2. Supporting Reasons. "I know this because . . ."
3. Emotion. "So now I feel . . ."

Always use a MOI immediately after clearing the ISE to validate and anchor all the changes. Then, as you grow the Child up through the SSEs, you can take a moment to bring closure to the event before moving onto the next SSE. In this way, you can encourage integration incrementally.

In the ISE, when the client has finished the MOI, give the instruction to, "Find a place next to your heart where the little one can go and always feel your love." Before growing the Child up, give it a safe place to grow up in. You can place the client's hand over their heart or instruct them to place the Child there. This anchors the suggestion that the Child is now accepted as a Part of the client.

Once the Child has been accepted into the client's heart, give the suggestion, "And because she's there next to you heart, she can always remember (read through the list of positive insights, self-affirming suggestions, etc. generated by the client during the session.)"Then add, "So, she can always know that you deeply and completely love and accept her. As a result, *you* get to know that *you* are loved, and feel that way too. Isn't that nice?"

Bi-lateral hug.
To complete the process, instruct Adult to hug the Child and notice how good that feels. You can make this a kinesthetic experience by physically crossing the client's arms across their chest, Pharaoh style. The client can then give themselves a bi-lateral hug while Grownup says some parting words to the Child before moving on from the scene into the next SSE. This can be done silently or out loud.

As you grow the Child up through the SSEs, test to make sure that the event is clear. Then wrap up the event with a MOI. If you have time, you can even transfer the changes to the Adult by having the Child say to Grownup, "I've changed. As I change, you change. Because I *am*[35] you."

Again, test the results. Verify the acceptability of the suggestion by saying to the Adult, "You *have* changed, haven't you." (Notice that this is delivered as a statement, not a question.)

Once Adult verifies the change, repeat the Moment of Insight process with Adult saying, "I have changed. I know I have changed because (fill in the blank) ... So now I feel (fill in the blank)." This is a powerful way to compound change as it is occurring. The insights accrued by facilitating a series of Moments of Insight can then be used during your session wrap up to turn whatever happened in the session into a revelation for the client. But to utilize a moment of insight effectively, you need to keep good notes as you guide the client through the healing process. This ensures that the suggestions you deliver are completely acceptable because they have been verified and come directly from the client[36].

Mental Rehearsal/Future Pacing Techniques

The subconscious mind does not discriminate between real and imagined. When the client can imagine a situation or event without any resistance, this increases his resourcefulness and optimism toward

---

[35] The two most powerful words a person can say in the privacy of their own Mind are "I am." Use them wisely.
[36] Learn more in Ditch the Script: Get Everything You Need from the Client for Successful Hypnotherapy and Set Up to Wrap Up with Results. Available on Amazon.

the therapy as well as their future. Mental Rehearsal and Future Pacing are imagery exercises that can be used as both preliminary and polishing techniques. As preliminary techniques, they serve as uncovering techniques. As polishing techniques, they can be used to test the results and encourage a deeper level of integration.

Mental Rehearsal is a process where you have the client imagine a scene that would normally cause some discomfort. Because you are working with an imagined event, Mental Rehearsal can be used as a preliminary technique to reduce resistance to "going there." For example, going for blood tests, public speaking. As a polishing technique, it gives you a way to test the results and clean up any residual aspects.

Future Pacing is a process where the client moves forward in time. Like Mental Rehearsal, the client is imagining a situation, but this situation is in the future. It could be an anticipated event or simply a created scene. Used as a preliminary technique, Future Pacing can give you a look-see into what the client's subconsciously held beliefs are with respect to the presenting issue. As a polishing technique, it gives you a way to test the results and ensure the releasing process is complete.

Pay attention to the client's body language as he describes the imagined event(s). Any tension, tightness, or emotional triggering indicates that there is something still unresolved. In this case, the unresolved aspect can be amplified and Bridged off of, or noted for future work in session.

When an issue is truly resolved, both processes give the client the opportunity to feel proud by mentally experiencing what it's like to finally be in control of some aspect of their life. For example:

- feeling calm while speaking in public
- going out to dinner and making healthy food choices
- being around smokers and feeling sorry for them
- attending a family reunion and feeling safe and comfortable
- looking and feeling good in jeans or wedding dress

Pro-Regression Technique

Future Pacing shows you the client's expectations for the future. This gives you an effective testing technique by allowing you to identify unresolved aspects which may point to another ISE. Pro-Regression[37] is a variation on Future Pacing that gives you another way to find a Bridge to the ISE.

You can also use Pro-Regression with clients who are apprehensive about going back to painful events in their past. Instead of going back in time, you invite the client to move forward into an imagined future. Because it's "just imagination," there's no resistance to "going there." Because the client still has "the problem," there's a good chance that they are going to bump into it in their imagined future. When that happens, find the feeling and follow it back to the event responsible for causing it.

Step 1: Find it.
Find the emotion triggered by imagining the future event. That feeling is a Bridge to the event that caused it! It's a signal from the past.

---

[37] Jure Biechonski, School of Analytical and Cognitive Hypnotherapy International

Step 2: Feel it.

Make sure you have a strong Bridge by encouraging the client to feel the feeling fully. Then it's business as usual - regress and release. Follow the signal back to the ISE and release it where it got started.

Step 3: Heal it.

Release and validate. Release and validate. Release and validate. This incremental approach will restore clarity and balance to the mind-body system. As a result, the client will feel calmer and more relaxed, allowing insights to come to conscious awareness. Gather up these newer, better awareness' and carry them forward – back to the future.

Step 4: Seal it.

Replay the future scene to test the results. If there's still a block, repeat the process. Wash, rinse and repeat.

Grey Room Technique

The Grey Room is a multi-purpose imagery exercise that symbolizes the client's subconscious mind. You can use it as a diagnostic technique, a polishing technique, and a scenario for Chair Therapy.

As a diagnostic technique, you can have the client enter the Grey Room to identify key aspects which are connected with their presenting issue. As a polishing technique, you can use it at the end of a session or healing program to test for residual aspects and integrate change more fully.

Step 1: Set Up

To setup for the Grey Room, begin by having your clients imagine themselves in a grey, round room shaped like an igloo. The walls of the room are curved, and the room has a domed ceiling.

Next, direct the client to notice the walls. On the walls are little bits of what appear to be paper. They're like post-it notes. Some of these bits of paper are red and some of them are white. The red bits contain all the negative thoughts and uncomfortable feelings inside. All the negative, depressing, self-defeating, thought and emotional energies are stored in this room on the red bits of paper.

Next, have the client notice that, in the center of the room, there is a hole about 8" wide. Inform the client that he can pull down the red bits of paper, scrunch them up, and put them into the hole in the center of the room. As these bits are placed into the hole, they are sucked away, and dissolved into nothingness. Let the client know that it doesn't take very long. In just a few trips, he can gather up handfuls of the red post-it notes and dispose of them by putting them into the hole, where they dissolve away to nothingness.

As the old, negative, depressing, self-defeating thought and emotional energies are released and dissolved into nothingness, the positive, energizing, helpful thought and emotional energies held by the white bits of paper grow and expand to replace the red bits, filling the room with the color white.

As this happens, the client can feel healing and empowerment occurring as the old, uncomfortable feelings from the past are replaced with this warm, positive, cleansing, and revitalizing energy, the room fills with the color white.

Step 2: Release
Repeat these instructions. Then, give the client a period of silence to perform this task with instructions to let you know when they're done. Then, wait. Let the client do the work.

Step 3: Test

When the client reports that the task is complete, test. Instruct the client to check to *make sure* that all the red bits are completely gone. Suggest that there might be some hiding and to even check behind him, and under his feet. *Make sure there's nothing left.*

If the client discovers a red bit that won't release, the Grey Room now serves as a diagnostic technique. To use the Grey Room as a diagnostic technique, instruct the client to focus on that red bit and notice what word is written upon it. That word has everything to do with the client's issue! It's a block.

Instruct the client to focus on that word and find the feeling. Guide the client to name the emotion associated with that word, then use it to Bridge back to the causal event. Regress to the ISE and release the feelings trapped in that event. When the event is clear, come back into the Grey Room and pick up where you left off by making sure the room is completely clear of red bits.

Step 4: Integrate

When the client is *sure* that there is nothing left, that the room is now completely clear, the hole in the center of the room closes automatically. Now it's time to fill the void.

Bring the client's attention back to the white bits and the positive qualities that remain. Deliver suggestions to amplify the qualities associated with the color white. Really pour on the coals. Expand the energy of goodness.

Make sure the client is feeling it fully! Then, instruct the client to breathe in this healing color. As she breathes in the color white, continue pouring in the suggestions for all the desirable qualities associated with the color white. For example, enlightenment, encouragement, support, beauty, confidence, strength, self-belief, trust, worth, love, freedom, etc. Remember to include words that match the client's desired goal and benefits.

Make this a yummy experience! As the client continues to breathe in the positive qualities symbolized by white light, give the suggestion that the light is washing, and cleansing, and rinsing, and healing every part of him – mentally, physically, and emotionally. Encourage the client to allow this white light to fill him completely, saturating every muscle, nerve, fiber, tendon, bone, and every cell and atom of his being with this brighter, lighter, quality of feeling.

Direct Drive Technique

The Direct Drive Technique (DD) is a compounding technique developed by Gerald Kein of Omni-Hypnosis that uses autosuggestion and repetition to hammer in a new belief. This technique is commonly used to polish off a smoking cessation program by reinforcing the new identity of a non-smoker, but it can be adapted very easily to any issue.

You can use the Direct Drive Technique to compound any new belief, but it is especially effective for "I am" statements of identity.

Formulate a statement of belief. For example, "I am now a non-smoker; I'll be a non-smoker for the rest of my life." Then, instruct the client to repeat the suggestion, either out loud or in the privacy of her own mind.

Gerry Kein recommended that the statement be repeated a minimum of 15 times. Unfortunately, this can get very boring, so the tendency is to quit too soon. To prevent this, Gerry suggested making a recording that you can use for your smoking cessation programs. All you need to do is get the client started, then turn on the recording and let the client continue without you.

The key to success with Direct Drive Technique is emotion. As the client repeats the suggestion, encourage her to imagine it and feel it *as if* it were already true. Focused intent wins the prize! Give the suggestion that the more feeling is present, the more powerful the effect will be. Then, suggest that you're going to give the client a few minutes of privacy to really 'go for the gold'. Switch on the recording and leave the room. When you return, simply join in with the recording to take over, turn off the player, and continue with wrapping up your session.

Heart Breathing

Heart Breathing is a very gentle, calming exercise that focuses attention on the heart. Because it is so maternal, it makes a lovely polishing technique following Inner Child or Bereavement Work.

Once thought of as a pump, the heart is now recognized as one of three "brains" in the body – the head brain, heart-brain, and gut brain. Research indicates that all three brains are in communication with one another. The heart has a system of neurons that have both short and long-term memory, and their signals can affect our emotional experiences.

According to HeartMath Institute, the heart emits an electromagnetic field that can be measured up to several feet away from the body. This electromagnetic field changes according to our emotions. Negative emotions disrupt the nervous system of the body. Positive emotions result in a state of coherence. This generates physiological benefits such as boosting immune function (which begins in the gut). When a client accesses a positive state, you can use Heart Breathing to facilitate integration. It's really yummy for the client.

Just have the client focus on the positive feeling in or around the heart. It might be love, peace, safety, or well-being. Whatever the client is experiencing, validate it. This is healing.

Invite the client to make a soft fist and place it gently over her heart chakra/center of chest. Then, while breathing deeply into the heart, have the client slowly rotate her fist in a circular motion, gently rubbing the area of the heart. This feels very soothing and brings attention to the area of the heart. Another option is to slowly and gently pat the area next to the heart with the flat of the hand.

To amplify the feeling, ask the client what color the positive feeling might be. Invite her flow that color into her heart by breathing into the heart. Have her notice how that feeling expands within her. Continue to expand the energies from the heart throughout the body.

If there is a physical area of discomfort in the body, send that feeling/color into that specific area. Saturate every muscle nerve and fiber with the healing power of feeling/color. To make it even more powerful, use autosuggestion or direct suggestion to deliver suggestions of love and self-acceptance.[38]

---

[38] Abdominal breathing allows more oxygen to get to the muscles, allowing muscles to relax, relieving pain and stress. It also has a calming effect on the brain and nervous system.

Color Breathing Technique

Color Breathing[39] is a variation on progressive relaxation that is useful for physical or emotional disorders. Once the client has been guided through this process, she can easily repeat it on her own, so it's useful as homework for certain clients.

Here the client goes inside and intuits (sense, feel) what color or colors the body needs at this time. Once the color or colors have been identified, instruct the client to begin breathing in through the nose and out through the mouth. With each inhalation, the client imagines that color is coming in through the bottoms of her feet and rising through the body. In this way, the body is progressively filling with color from the bottom up.

With each inhalation, the color moves further up inside the body, filling the body with cleansing and healing qualities, and releasing blockages. With each exhalation, have the client imagine that she is blowing out any blocked pieces that have been released by the color. Give the suggestion that as the client is blowing out any blocked pieces, she may notice a bitter taste in her mouth. Or it might feel like she's spitting out tiny pieces of paper.

This process is very flexible and can be adapted to whatever time you have available. You can do rounds to address aspects or a specific purpose. Each time invite a new color in. For example, the first round might be used as a diagnostic to identify any blocked areas in the body. The next round might then focus on releasing the blocks. The final round would then focus on filling the void with a new color.

---

[39] Patti Conklin

Following the releasing process, have the client go inside and do a scan of the body to see if there is any place the color didn't go. Any place the color didn't go indicates a block. This block can then be released by identifying what specific color might be needed to clear it completely.

Once released, the next round might be to invite a color needed for cleansing and rinsing away any residual blockages.

The round after that might bring in an energizing color/energy to increase motivation or confidence, amplify calmness, or enhance the body's natural healing capabilities. What does the client need?

Finally, a color might be invited to seal in these changes and integrate them fully by expanding them out beyond the body. Color can be further expanded by sending it out into situations in the client's life in need of healing and transformation. It can be transmitted to loved ones, or to the planet as an act of unconditional love.

Be creative! The applications are limitless.

If a client reports that they had a disturbing dream between sessions, treat it as you would any triggering event. Invite the client to share their dream with you. Make sure the client uses present-tense language. That way, as they tell the Story, the client will be reliving the dream with you. The moment the client bumps into a feeling, you have a Bridge to the actual event responsible for creating that feeling. Focus on that feeling!

~ **The Devil's Therapy**: *Hypnosis Practitioner's Essential Guide to Effective Regression Hypnotherapy*

CHAPTER 12: BIG HAIRY-SCARY EVENT?

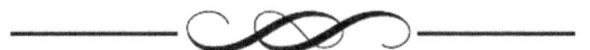

When an event is left unresolved, it's because whatever was happening was being perceived through a consciousness that lacked either the maturity or the resources needed to be able to cope with the situation. This generated uncomfortable feelings and emotions. That's what makes any event memorable – how it feels. ~ **The Devil's Therapy**

When the subconscious mind is willing to show you a painful event from the past, know that it trusts you to help it get some relief. But be prepared because discovering where the bodies are buried can mean that things are going to get very real, very fast. Be prepared for abreactions. No matter what is brought to the surface of consciousness, know that you're right where you need to be. All the client needs to do is follow your instructions and they'll get what they need.

The easiest way to process a traumatic event is to titrate it by conducting the uncovering, releasing, reframing and re-educating processes in rounds. Titrating an event is a process of uncovering and releasing one perception at a time. This prevents overwhelming (and re-traumatization) the client.

Recognize that this is what the subconscious mind has been protecting the client from. Allowing the uncovering process to occur in bite-size increments makes it safe for the client to allow more of the memory to come to conscious awareness. This approach also allows a more thorough clearing of all the contributing aspects.

Accruing increments of relief, in this way, will increase the client's confidence in the process, keeping them committed to achieving their Therapeutic Goal.

The Steps:

1. Preliminary uncovering process.
2. Reparent the Child.
3. Find the first feeling.
4. Find the thought.
5. Reality-check the thought.
6. Find the next feeling.
7. Re-story the event.

Step 1: Preliminary uncovering process.

What happened? Guide the client to step into the event, then conduct the preliminary uncovering process to get a general sense of what happened, where it happened, and who was involved in the event. You can help to reduce resistance by reminding the client that this is only a memory, there's nothing here that they haven't already lived through. It's just that the subconscious mind doesn't know this, yet. "We're here to change that so you can feel better."

Step 2: Reparent the Child.

Once the initial uncovering work is complete, the client's job is to reparent their Inner Child. This begins with expressing love and acceptance for the Child, then promising to be there for the Child from now on. This provides the Child with something that was missing during the original experience – a source of security. The client then prepares the Child for what is *about to happen* in the ISE.

Bringing in adult consciousness to educate and support the Child solves the most fundamental problem of any ISE - the Child had to deal with a distressing situation *alone*. Herein lies the key to transforming a traumatic experience in childhood. It's in uncovering how the Child is making sense of what's happening.

Everything will play out exactly as it did the first time. The only thing that changes is that the Child now knows that she will survive and grow up to adulthood. After all, Grownup is living proof of this. Adult consciousness is then present to provide what the Child most needed - love and support in making sense of the experience.

Step 3: Find the first feeling.
Rewind to the beginning and replay the event with the client giving you a report of what's happening. The moment the client bumps into an uncomfortable emotion, stop right there. Release the feeling. Get the pressure off and the client will have greater clarity with which to report.

Step 4: Find the thought.
Use autosuggestion to identify the thought that is responsible for generating that uncomfortable feeling. For example, "I feel (scared) because... (put an ending on it.)" This is how the Child is interpreting what's happening. Is that thought true?

Step 5: Reality-check the thought.
Reality check that thought with Grownup. If it's not true, re-educate the Child about what *is* true. For example, the Child thinks that Mom

is abandoning her. She thinks Mom is never going to come back. That's generating fear. But the truth is that Mom is dropping the Child off at daycare for the first time. Mom's only going to be gone for a few hours. The Child can now feel safe and realize there are other children to play with.

If it's true, the next step is to help the client come to acceptance. It happened. It wasn't the greatest experience. But it's a foul wind that doesn't blow any good, and every cloud has a silver lining. What could the Child learn from this experience that would serve her in future? What's the nugget of wisdom, the gift in the garbage?

Step 6: Find the next feeling.
Once you have cleared both the thought and feeling, rewind and replay the event until the client bumps into the next uncomfortable feeling. Repeat the steps until the client can move through the entire event without getting triggered.

Step 7: Re-story the event.
Re-storying is the process of transforming the narrative about what happened in the ISE, how it affected the client, and how it developed into a life story as it evolved through the SSEs. But you can't just rewrite a memory. You have to transform it by changing how it *feels*. The way to transform how a memory feels is to help the Child get through the event without being negatively impacted by it.

The client's story has power. It defines them. It decides what they can expect in the future because of those past experiences. As a result, it is creating their reality NOW. Changing the beginning of the story changes the client's overall lens on life. As a result, the SSEs will automatically transform.

Identify the unmet needs of the Child in the event. Then, change the meaning that experience was given. First, identify how the Child is interpreting the experience. What meaning is the Child giving to what's happening? Then, ask Adult Consciousness to reality-check these thoughts. Ask, "Is that true?"

If the Child's interpretation of the situation is not accurate, invite Grownup to tell the Child the truth about what's happening. Ask, "What does the Child most need to know to get through the event feeling okay?" or "If you'd known then, what you know now, how might that have changed things?" Providing the Child with this information removes the initial shock of the ISE.

If the Child's interpretation of what's happening is true, what's needed is acceptance and forgiveness. In this case, validate the perceptions and feelings of the Child. Then find a way to bring the client to a place of recognition. It happened. It's sad but true. And while it wasn't the greatest experience, *it's over*. Help the client to realize that the past is the past. This allows the Subconscious Mind to finally relax. That's when healing happens.

Troubleshooting Trauma

Client Abreacts?

When a client abreacts, recognize this response as the subconscious mind expressing a need. It's doing exactly what it was designed to do. The problem is that the subconscious mind doesn't know that the cause of that uncomfortable feeling is in the past. The purpose of regression work is to put the past in the past by working *with* the subconscious mind. Get it working with you.

If the client abreacts, ask, "True or false – you're aware of what's happening." If the client says, "True," quickly uncover the Story then move the Child to a safe place such as "before anything bad happens."

Hysterical abreaction?
Get the client to safety. You can use Gerry Kein's Nine Magic Words to temporarily remove the client from the perceived threat. "The scene fades, and you grow peaceful with your breathing."

Wait until the client has restabilized, then return to reviewing the event. This ensures that you don't reinforce the client's learned avoidance strategies and keeps the client responsible for the result. For example, "Now we are going to go back again. This time you are going to get the rest of those emotions out. You are in control at all times, but you like the thought of just getting them out. You already realize how good it's going to feel to get them out."

Return to the beginning of the scene and run the event again.

Child is frozen or numb?
Situations of severe trauma such as witnessing violence or being subjected to abuse can cause dissociation. If the Child is frozen, numb, unable to speak, or witnessing what's happening from outside the body, what's happening in the situation is overwhelming the nervous system of the body. Dissociating gives them a way out of the situation.

Dissociation is not the problem. Dissociation is a Child's natural coping mechanism. If it's too much for the Child, get them out. The client doesn't have to relive a terrifying past experience from the past. You just need to know what's happening to generate that big hairy-scary feeling so you can release it.

If the subconscious mind takes the client into a Big Hairy-Scary event, take charge, and provide safety. Let the client know that everything is under control. Reassure them that you know what to do, that you've "got this." Say, "Your subconscious mind has just shown us what's calling for healing so let yourself stay focused on that feeling."

Child is experiencing terror?

If the Child is experiencing intense fear, provide some distance from the perceived source of fear. This will allow you to safely process the event without retraumatizing the client. For example, if the Child is feeling terrified, place the Child safely in the background while you have a talk with Grownup. Say, "(Child) can't hear us. True or false – you're aware of what's happening." This will allow you to uncover a general sense of what's happening to cause the Child's feelings of overwhelm.

Adult consciousness can provide what the Child needs to move through the event without feeling overwhelmed. What the Child most needed, the first time, was support. She needed help in making sense of what was happening. She needed to know that what was happening would end and that she was going to survive. She needs to know that, while uncomfortable, it won't last forever, and that she is learning important lessons that will empower her later in life.

What else does the Child need? Ask Grownup because there's no real separation between the Child and Grownup. She knows.

Grownup shocked?

If what's happening in the event came as a shock to the conscious mind of the client (i.e. Grownup), don't make the mistake of trying to proceed with a frightened Child *and* an unstable Grownup!

Your priority is to make it safe for the Child to face what happened in that shocking event. You need a Grownup to do that. Prepare your client to step in and be a loving support for their younger self.

Option 1: Instruct the (adult) client to drift up to a safe distance above the scene. From this safe vantage point, they can review the event with the understanding that it is "just a memory," it's in the past, and they are a grownup, now. This provides sufficient emotional distance from the experience to allow you to conduct the preliminary uncovering process to find out what happened, who was involved, and how it ended.

Guide the adult to release any triggered emotions and restore balance. Then, in a matter-of-fact tone say something like, "Well, now we know what we're dealing with. Realize that this situation in the past – it's just a memory. You've already lived through it, once. The problem is that (Child) doesn't know that. As a result, your subconscious has been stuck in that event, trying to find a way out. We can change that. Are you ready? This is where your miracle lies. In a moment, I'm going to count from three down to one. At the count of one find yourself right *before* the event. So, nothing bad has happened yet, understand?"

You're now set up to guide the client to step into the event and be with the Child. From there, you can switch back and forth between Child consciousness and adult consciousness. Conduct the reparenting process, then have Grownup prepare the Child for what's going to happen. Before running the event, verify that the Child understands and believes Grownup.

Option 2: Because the traumatic event is a source of distress for the Child, the client is vulnerable to triggering. Remember, they share the same feelings. This makes what happened *after* the traumatic experience just as important as what happened during the trauma. For example, did help eventually come? Go immediately after the event to the point where "it's over". Find out what happened in hindsight. Then, provide support in releasing the emotions attached to "what just happened" using past-tense language.

If the child had to endure the aftermath of the experience alone, bringing in adult consciousness to provide love and support will change the impact that experience had on the client.

Release the emotional charge until the client can speak calmly about "that experience." Then, bring in Grownup to conduct the hypnoanalysis process so that you can uncover the information needed to help prepare the Child for the event. For example, what does the Child need to know to get through this experience without being traumatized by it? What does the adult client *wish* she had known? If she had known that *before* it happened, how might it have changed things?

Had the client known then, what she knows *now* - that she was going to get through it, that she'd survive, that she would get to grow up - would it have been so *bad*? If the client says, "yes," identify the specific "bad" aspects and continue releasing until the client can accept the truth of how it was.

The goal is for the client to realize that, had she known how the event was going to end, in advance, the big, hairy-scary event wouldn't have been so bad. This gives you a client who is ready to prepare the Child and participate in the Inner Child Work. Once the client realizes that, had she known what she knows now, the event wouldn't have come as such a shock, the next step is to gain permission to review the event to heal it. For example, "With that in mind, would you be willing to go back to immediately before anything bad happens and *prepare the Child for what's going to happen* . . . because, if the Child knows what you know - that she gets to grow up - it changes everything for the better. Your whole life changes for the better. Would you be willing to do that so you can heal?"

This is a Contract. The client is agreeing to do the work necessary to self-heal. Once the agreement is established, guide the client back to before anything happens. Remind the Adult that nothing has happened, yet. The Child doesn't know what's going to happen. It's Adult's job to prepare the Child for what's *going* to happen.

Option 3: Titrate the event. Don't try to process the entire event at once. Titrating is an analytical technique that allows you to process one small measure of perception, thought, feeling or emotion at a time. Chunking down, in this way, makes it safer to allow the undigested pieces of a painful experience to be reviewed, and released one small bite at a time. Much easier.

Think 'increments of change'. For example, the moment something feels like it's too much for the Child, give the command, "Everything stops." You can then focus on releasing the energy attached to that specific perception, thought, feeling or emotion.

Slowing things down and working on smaller pieces of a traumatic experience puts an end to the overwhelm, allowing the client to come back into balance. Once balance has been restored, you can move forward to the next critical moment.

Option 4: Providing some distance and chunking down how much information needs to be processed in any given moment can significantly reduce the client's arousal.

If something is happening that the client doesn't want to look at, or is too triggering for the client, give the client control over how much is revealed.

Install a protective barrier such as a glass wall or a one-way mirror which allows the client to view the scene while giving you a report about what's happening. You can even suggest that the glass is fogged with steam. The client can then clear a small peephole through which to view what's happening[40]. This gives the client some control over how much is revealed to them.

Adult is resistant to supporting Child?
When the client rejects their Inner Child, recognize that this is self-rejection. Unfortunately, now you have a bigger problem to deal with because adult consciousness is contaminating the original event. You need a Grownup to do the Inner Child Work because the Child is already traumatized. This is one mess that can be prevented by taking the time to assess the client's readiness *before* guiding them back to painful events in childhood. Train your client to be a loving support to their Inner Child before "going there."

If you still have a problem, regress back to where the Child deserves only love and acceptance. Then, focus on educating the Adult client on what *every* Child needs and deserves.

Client tries to change the ISE?
Releasing changes how the client feels. As a result, they may try to change the story. For example, a client releases the fear associated with an event of abuse. When you rewind and replay the event, he

---

[40] Many thanks to Wally Mueller, Advanced Hypnosis, Calgary, Alberta for this technique!

experiences anger. Anger is more empowering than fear. As a result, he reports hitting or kicking the Offender. This, however, is not what happened. It's what the client *wishes* had happened.

The problem with this is that the subconscious mind never forgets. The original memory is still there. Creating a false memory will generate an internal conflict. You can still use it, though. You just need to remove it before wrapping up the session.

When the client tries to change what happened in an event, let them. Don't interrupt. Just let them have that experience. When they have satisfied that need, say, "But that's not how it happened, is it?" Once you have cancelled the fantasy, ask, "What does Child need to know to get through that situation without being negatively affected in any way?"

Always tell the Child the truth. Do not minimize. Do not reinforce avoidance strategies. The Child survived. Grownup is proof of the Child's ability to get through the most challenging experience. All that's needed is for the Adult to prepare the Child to meet the trouble.

Make the client responsible for the results. The answers are within. What does the Child need? Find a way to provide it. Educate the Child. Once the Child has the understanding needed, rewind and replay the event the way it happened the first time. This time through, the client will be further empowered by facing the facts about what happened without experiencing any emotional distress.

Providing what was needed the first time turns the ISE into an opportunity to develop resilience. Releasing the emotional charge results in a state of calm relaxation and clarity. This heightened state of awareness is wide open to accepting positive suggestions which reinforce the changes which have occurred. They have successfully overcome a challenge! This changes everything! When you grow the Child up through the SSEs, this wiser, more empowered way of being in the world will grow and develop with them.

Remember, the healing lies in the Child's ability to get through the ISE without being negatively impacted by it. This can't happen if you change what happened. The only thing that needs to change is the Child's interpretation of that experience. Then you can transform it into a source of empowerment for the client. For this to happen, the Child needs to learn something of value from that experience. This will allow the Child go grow up feeling good about himself by knowing what the Adult didn't know the first time.

Client goes to womb?
When the client returns to the womb, they may not know where they are. This is because the infant's perceptions are primarily sensation. The client may feel like she's floating or, if it's close to delivery time, "tight."

Client goes to birth experience?
The contractions that occur during the birthing process put pressure on the infant which can be frightening. Impressions of being unwanted, unloved, or hurting Mom are common causes of hurt and fear associated with birth.

With any pre-verbal event, whether in the womb, during birth, or following birth, it is important to help the infant separate her feelings from Mom's feelings. This will restore the child's ability to feel safe and secure.

Difficult births, necessitating the use of forceps or Caesarian Section, are traumatizing to the Child. In this case, the infant is frightened, not only for herself, but for Mom, as well. Even standard medical procedure such as cutting the umbilical cord or taking the Child away to be suctioned and cleaned, following delivery, can be interpreted as life-threatening to a helpless infant. This is traumatizing because the Child has never been away from Mom. For example, during my own regression to birth, I experienced what it's like to have the umbilical cord cut too soon. One moment I was comfortable, safe and warm. The next moment, an abrupt jolt went through my entire body. I froze in terror! That moment of separation is trauma.

A Case of Birth Trauma

What motivated Alice to come for hypnotherapy was a desire to go on a vacation. The problem was that she was afraid to fly, afraid to ride an escalator, elevator or enter any closed-in place. Even sitting in the back seat of a car caused her to panic. That meant that taxis were out! Alice had missed her sister's wedding because the reception was held in a hotel. The long hallways terrified Alice and sent her running for safety. She had been to a psychiatrist who used Cognitive Behavioral Therapy (CBT) to help her to cope with elevators, but she still had the fear.

Regression revealed complications during her birth. Alice got stuck in the birth canal and, for what seemed like an eternity, was trapped. She felt pressure all around her. She could also feel Mom's fear. While she was soon brought into the world, a healthy infant, no one knew that those few moments of oxygen deprivation had caused epilepsy. The seeds of her claustrophobia had also been planted.

Following release of the birthing trauma, we were able to test the results. At the time, I had a little two-door sports car. The back seat was really very constricting, so I asked Alice if she thought getting in there would cause her any discomfort. She said that normally it would but she was willing to try. I then opened the driver's door and invited her to sit in the back seat. I assured her that I would leave the door open, but I wanted to test to see if she was completely clear.

Alice got into the back seat and within moments her eyes were wide as saucers. "Nothing!" she exclaimed. "I could never have done this!"

"That's great!" I smiled, putting the driver's seat back. "How do you feel now?" She laughed a little nervously, then realized she was still okay. "Nothing! I don't believe this!" Alice exclaimed.

I then climbed into the driver's seat and, upping the ante, closed the door. "Still nothing."

I then started the engine. "Let's take a little spin up the road, okay?"

"Sure!" Alice smiled. I drove to the end of the road and, looking in the rear-view mirror, saw a grinning Alice with both fists raised in victory. "Yes!"

If a client goes back to birth, *stay there*. There's so much involved at birth that you can treat it like an ISE. It likely is for something! If you're in the birth scene, the client has a second chance to get started on the right foot in life. By allowing her younger self to move forward into a safer, more loving world, she is 'paying it forward.' Not only will this reduce the charge in subsequent events, if the client's mother is still alive, their relationship will mysteriously improve. I kid you not.

Once the event is clear, and the Child can go through the experience without any distress, guide her to forgive everyone. That includes Mom, the doctor, the nurses, and anyone else who was present. Don't forget Dad. Whether he was present at the birth, waiting outside, or somewhere else, he needs to be forgiven. There's no need to have a reason to forgive anyone.

Always get forgiveness toward Mom. She's the most important person in the Child's Life. Subconsciously, Mom is Source. She's God-in-the-flesh. Many of our life-long issues are linked to our relationship with our mother. Have the child look deeply into Mom's eyes and tell you what she notices. There are two reasons for doing this.

First, eye contact is integral to bonding. Failure to adequately bond is a key contributor to sensitizing a person to trauma.

Second, making eye contact will help facilitate a deep level of forgiveness toward Mom.

When the child looks deeply into Mom's eyes, if she finds love, amplify it for all its worth. Let the client get filled up with that Love. If the client is spiritual, you can compound that love further by bringing in the Love of the Universe. If she looks into Mom's eyes and doesn't feel connected for whatever reason, there's a block. Focus on releasing that feeling. Then reframe using the following technique.

A Case of Abuse

The client presented with BIG emotions. He was going through a crisis in a relationship that had thrown him into the emotional blender. He was terrified that the relationship was going to end and that he would be left alone - again. He was angry with himself because he was failing in yet another relationship. He was profoundly sad. His feelings were bubbling up to the surface. He recognized that these feelings had haunted him for most of his life. As a result, he was serious about creating change, willing to commit to a process of self-healing, and ready to allow feelings and emotions to be part of the healing process.

First session: Age 2, Angry Relative
Client regressed spontaneously to age two with an angry relative. After conducting the ISE test, we Bridged back further to age one with Mom being neglectful. Throughout the process the client was experiencing lots of physical sensations. Both events boiled down to fear of somebody else's anger. This became the client's fear of his own anger. As a result, he was very resistant to recognizing or allowing his own anger.

To his credit, he managed to get three or four rounds of releasing anger into the pillow. Then, he retreated. I switched to tapping on releasing his resistance to allowing anger to be felt and expressed. This cleared the resistance allowing the events at age one and two to be cleared. This resulted in significant relief for the client. At the start of the session, the client couldn't say the words "I accept myself". By the session wrap-up, he could easily say "I deeply and completely *love* and accept myself" - and feel it.

During the post-hypnosis debriefing, he revealed that Mom had been "violent and angry." I made a note of this for when it came time to do the Forgiveness Work.

Second session: Age 3, Dad's Disapproval (Anger)
The second session was just three days later when the client was plunged into another wave of emotional overwhelm by another dose of criticism from his girlfriend. He spontaneously regressed to age

three, this time to deal with the perception of Dad's disapproval which generated fear, shame, and loneliness. This event held many layers and, again, lots of physical sensations. Clearing the event resulted in the client giving himself permission to open to love. Real love. True love.

Unfortunately, the client was still under the illusion that "real" love is manic, head-over-heels, lose-yourself-in-another blissful attachment and, consequently, a state of being wide open to hurt. But the feeling he described as "opening" and "love flooding in" was healing. I allowed the client a few minutes to marinate in the good feelings associated with these shifts before wrapping up the session.

Third session: Age 3, Neighbor Boys (Fear)
Following the second session, the client went off to visit family for a couple of weeks. When he returned, he was 'three-bags-full' of feeling bad accompanied by a new realization that his "family is really messed up!" Rather than jumping into the therapeutic process at the first sign of tension or tears, I let the client talk.

The more the client talked about stuff, the more his discomfort grew. He started to choke up. This time, the feeling was "lonely." When offered the Sentence Stem to complete, "I feel lonely because …" the client offered, "There's no one to feel my good feelings with!" Beautiful! A couple of releasing rounds followed with the focus on the lonely feeling in the body. This helped to restore the client's confidence in the process. Once he experienced some relief, I asked the client if "that feeling" was a new feeling or and old, familiar feeling. The client blubbered in response, "MY WHOLE LIFE!"

This statement was complimented with a nice, big fat abreaction. Awesome! I gave the command, "stay focused on that "my whole life feeling in your stomach" and counted him back to an earlier time. The feeling bridged back to age three. Mom was chastising the neighbor boys causing the Child to feel tight in his stomach. Really tight. The tight feeling was soon identified as "scared."

Sentence Stems on "I feel scared because …" was completed with "I froze"" This is trauma.[41] Immediately, I slowed things down and focused on releasing the fear associated with the feeling of the body freezing up.

For a 3-year-old, the sensations of the freeze response are terrifying. The problem is that there wasn't anything happening in the scene to indicate the presence of a threat. Nor was there anything preventing the Child from fleeing from the perceived threat. Something must have happened *before* this moment in time, something that would make the 3-year-old Child *know* to freeze in response.

Following the release of the fear anchored to the freeze response, the client's Mind spontaneously regressed to a scene just prior to Mom chastising the boys. It was the same event but just prior to the fear coming on. I won't share details, here, but it was an experience of sexual abuse. The physical sensations trapped in this event were BIG - doubling over, groaning, severe knot-pain in the guts. There were lots of layers trapped in that moment in time including fear of not knowing what's going on, fear of being alone, fear that no one is there to help.

---

[41] There are two books I highly recommend. "Making Sense of Suffering" by Stettbacher and "The Body Bears the Burden" by Scaer. Stettbacher's book clearly shows how the body clamping down becomes a learned response which results in suffering. Dr. Scaer's book shows how our biological programming to release feelings, naturally, gets over-ridden by our thinking mind, locking the energy into the body. When we perceive a threat, our fight or flight response kicks in. When we can't fight or flee, we freeze.

Bingo! Fear of being alone was the client's presenting issue! Below "that fear" was shame and self-blame because the Child decided, "I did it." The thought, "It's my fault" brought up more fear. Then, the thought came, "I'll be alone the rest of my life."

Boom. This was the underlying cause. That decision, based in the cognitive and emotional maturity of the Child, was an absolute. This is what was responsible for the client's presenting problem as an adult.

In a way, a single event has its own timeline. It's a story with a beginning, middle, and end. *Before* this event, the Child was feeling good – safe, happy, okay. Then, something happened to change that. What happened made him feel vulnerable, powerless and frightened. The ending of this story permanently altered his perception of himself, others, and life. Several reviews of the event followed to release all the contributing aspects.

The process of repeatedly rewinding and replaying the event resulted in greater clarity. Suddenly, the client realized, "that this wasn't the first time." The devil is in the details. With the internal stress associated with this traumatic experience significantly reduced, the Child feeling much better. As a result, he had sufficient clarity to report what, exactly, was going on. The Child had experienced this before. It wasn't a new experience! I asked the Child, "How many times has this happened."

Without hesitation the Child reported, "This is the third time." When you're three-years-old, you may not be sure what your age is, but you know how many times you've had to endure physical and emotional abuse. I suggested that he take us back to the "first time." I was hopeful that we'd be able to go directly the ISE. The subconscious, however, had other plans and promptly took us back to the second event. Damn!

The ISE had yet to be revealed. The third event (SSE) had to do with Mom chastising the neighbor boys. The second event (SSE) also involved the neighbor boys. Here's what happened. The neighbor boys took the 3-year-old inside their fort while making the Child's older siblings wait outside. It was dark inside the fort. The Child felt very isolated and alone. This seeded his fear of being alone.

I guided the client to release a significant amount of internal pressure, then, rather than dwelling on the pain and abuse, I shot for the ISE. Here's why. The client had released a tremendous amount of pressure and was feeling the relief. He reported that there were three events and that this was the second. One more bounce and I would have the causal event. If I could clear the ISE, the SSEs would be much easier for the client to face. The client would be more equipped to face those later events because they wouldn't come as a surprise.

I counted him back to the first time. "3,2, 1, be there. Say, Here I am … and I feel …." The client reported, "Numb."

CH: "Does it feel like its daytime or nighttime?"

Child: "I don't know."

CH: "That's okay. Does it seem like its light or dark?"

Child: "Light … I think it's daytime."

CH: "Good. Are you inside or outside?"

Child: "Inside the house."

CH: "Good. You know where your Mind has you. Does it feel like you're alone or with someone?"

Child: "The house is quiet. I'm alone?"

CH: "How young might you be that you're alone in the house when it's quiet?"

Child: "Three. I'm Three."

CH: "Where is everyone that you're Three, alone in the house?"

Child: "I think maybe they're sleeping.... I'm in Mom and Dad's room."

CH: "Good. Say, "Here I am. / I'm Three / alone inside the house / it's quiet / and I feel (put an end on it.)"

Child: "Numb."

CH: "That's okay. When we're little, we don't always know how to feel all our feelings. Where do you feel that numb feeling in your body?"

Child: "All over." (Freeze response!)

Because there was resistance (fear) to uncovering the details of the event, I kept the client focused on the feelings in the body. I have found that if you keep releasing the pressure, the details will surface on their own. There is no need to push.

It took several rounds to break through the numbness because the client kept associating to his current pain with the girlfriend. He was 'connecting the dots' but it was too soon for that. Instead, I pulled him back into the scene for another round of releasing by saying, "That's okay. Your subconscious mind is connecting the dots. You stay focused on that feeling at three years old."

Like ogres, traumatic experiences have layers. These layers included:

Scared because . . . "I'll be like this forever."

Scared because . . . "It's not safe to feel my feelings."

Scared because . . . "It's not safe to feel anger!"

Notice how these are three different fears? The thought causes the feeling. The thought, "It's not safe" generates "that fear" while the thought, "I'll be stuck in this pain forever" is the cause of another fear.

At some point, the client slid right out of the chair and onto the floor! He was literally howling. *Really loud!* (Someone from the unit next door actually came over and banged on the front door to see if I was okay.)

We go where we need to go to get the healing, so I got down on the floor next to the client and continued offering suggestions of encouragement while pulling out my futon bolster pillow. I was just thankful that I'd worn pants that day and made a note to myself - from now on, skirts and dresses are for presentations. Session work requires yoga gear!

A futon is very dense and heavy. Because it is very strong and solid, it's ideal for pounding out strong emotions like anger. A bolster is shaped like a tube. This is the perfect shape for pounding out painful emotions because the client can put it between his legs. It's like a mini-punching bag. Remember, the goal is to release the trapped emotions by pumping them into the pillow. This gives the feeling a place to go. It's not about hitting, punching or any expression of violence which will only reinforce the fear.

The client *pumped* the anger, fear, and pain of unresolved grief into the pillow. Wave after wave of emotion was released into the pillow. With each release, I guided the client to validate the increment of change. When the fear was gone, we moved onto putting the *remaining* anger into the pillow. The more anger the client released, the better he felt, but the cause of "that anger" was not yet clear. It took a while to get to the "because" behind "that anger." I just kept encouraging the client to put it into the pillow while saying, "I feel angry! / I'm allowed to feel angry! /I'm allowed to put it in the pillow! /I'm allowed to feel it all! / All my feelings are good /even the angry ones! /I keep going until it's all gone!/ etc."

To my amazement he kept going! He'd stop briefly to rest during which time I would deliver suggestions to compound the changes that were occurring. Then, we'd go back to releasing the feeling into the pillow. Eventually, he came to sufficient clarity to recognize, "I feel angry because . . ." The thought behind "that anger" was, *The world is unfair. I hurt all the time.*

Boom. That's a belief that's based in the thoughts of a Child. As Angeles Arrien[42] says, *"That's* a dream that doesn't have to happen!"

Child: "I hurt all the time."

CH: "I hurt because …."

Child: "It hurts to hold my feelings in!" (This came as an insight to the client.)

---

[42] Cultural anthropologist and author of The Four Fold Way: Walking the Paths of the Warrior, Healer, Teacher and Visionary.

CH: "That's right. Say, I'm learning. (Validate and reframe) I'm learning to feel all my feelings. / All my feelings are good. / Even the bad ones. / Good ones, bad ones, / big ones, small ones. / fat ones, skinny ones, / bald ones, hairy ones. (Laughter brings release) / I'm allowed to feel ALL my feelings. / These are MY feelings. / I'm allowed to feel them / because if I can feel it, I can heal it. / The only place they can hurt me is trapped inside. / I know that now / because I let myself feel them / and NOW I feel …"

Client: "Really great!"

When the anger was spent, we compounded the client's recognition that he was feeling better, was allowed to feel better, was looking forward to feeling better "just knowing that I made it through." I then added, "Even the PILLOW made it through!" (Humor is great as a follow-up for catharsis.) By this time, the client had been flopping around on the floor of my session room for well over an hour. Even though he was feeling massive relief, waves of grief were starting to come up. This was not the time to end the session. Grief needs to be heard. As a result, talking is an effective way to release it so I guided the client to tap while he talked.

As he talked, he cried softly, tenderly. I gently affirmed, "That's okay. You're feeling your truest feelings. You're allowed to feel all your feelings. That's what allows you to feel better. Go inside your body – tell me what you notice *now* …"

The client reported feeling good, relaxed, and *really tired*. Following a major release, the client will often report feeling tired. Reframe this by saying, "True or false – you feel *relaxed*." This suggestion will often be met with surprise as the client realizes that what they are really feeling is relaxation.

Relaxation is a natural by-product of releasing the internal pain and pressure associated with trapped emotions. It's a letting go. Once this happens, use a statement of validation by instructing the client to say, "It's over. I can finally relax."

In this case, the client indicated that there was another layer trying to claw its way to the surface. But 2 ½ hours of releasing work is enough. Rome wasn't built in a day. Neither was the problem. And moving mountains can take time. This was the perfect place to button things up for the next session.

Post-Hypnotic Debriefing

The client indicated that he was planning to have another talk with his girlfriend that night. But what he had in mind was some variation on, "Come back, there's a part of my heart you haven't stomped on yet!" Clearly, we weren't done, yet. So, I gently suggested, "You might want to go home and just relax, tonight. Give yourself time to rest and recalibrate. After all, you've done a lot of releasing. And you know that's true! Your body is allowed to rest and relax and recalibrate. Maybe have a nice hot bath, listen to some soothing music, do some self-hypnosis … just enjoy some ALONE time…"

He decided to cancel his plans with the girlfriend. (Good call, buddy!) He then did a little reflecting on his family of origin and realized, "Life is a struggle" was the family program. He agreed that this belief was worth getting rid of. He was still lying on the floor as we continued to talk about how all this "stuff" had been locked up inside of him since he was three years old, and how internal stress and pressure builds up over time, and how all those feelings had been stacking up on him, and how the current situation with his girlfriend had acted as a trigger. Suddenly, he got it. With red, weepy eyes, he exclaimed, "OH MY

GAWD! I can actually SEE him! For the first time I can SEE him!" With release comes greater clarity. The client could clearly see the Child that he once was. Prior to this, he had only a felt-sense. He was so surprised by this new sense that he got teary, again.

I instructed him to gently close his eyes and, as he could now see the Child, to say, "I *found* you!" These are powerful words for the Child to hear. He then told the Child, "You matter to me," and "Your feelings brought me back to you," and "I deeply and completely love and accept you," and "Now that I've found you, *you'll never be alone again.*" Following this, the client realized that what he most needed was to spend time with his three-year-old self (reinforcing his decision to take some time alone tonight.) He then said that he was feeling very tired.

As this was my last client of the day, I wrapped him in a blanket, put a pillow under his head, set a glass of water next to him, and gave him permission to rest for as long as he needed. I then left him alone in the office to recover. After about 5 minutes, the client came out, looking bleary eyed but feeling grateful. He said that the feeling in his gut was still there, but that it was okay, that he could handle it. I suggested that he was now ready to start releasing stuff on his own. I gave him a tapping guide with the instructions, "If anything comes up between now and next session, you can get some relief. Realize there's only so much of that in there. You did good work today. You can feel it." We then scheduled the next session.

Subsequent Sessions

Subsequent sessions revealed that this client had grown up in an environment permeated by the anger of others. This terrified him as a child. Consequently, he learned to be terrified of his own anger.

Subsequent sessions focused on releasing all the anger that had gotten trapped inside. It took a lot of work to release his resistance to feeling "that feeling," but once achieved, he let 'er rip with the pillow - feathers flying!

Releasing anger consistently brought increasing insight. Realizing that it wasn't his fault resulted in self-forgiveness enabling him to begin to find some good in painful events of his past. The final breakthrough occurred in session five. Not surprisingly, the girlfriend issue had everything to do with Mom. However, the client skidded across the surface of that realization. It hadn't hit home, yet. It was too painful to face.

Facing the truth of one's past is not something that can be forced. It has to happen organically. As the Wicked Witch of the West stated, "These things must be handled delicately."[43] As more events of abuse were brought to light, it became increasingly evident that his subconscious mind had been protecting the client from the awareness of what had happened. But once the pressure was reduced sufficiently, the door opened spontaneously to the ISE.

The ISE Revealed

Three years old, again. This time, a beautiful, sunny day. The Child was feeling good, *really* good. Happy. His family had recently moved to a new place and life was exciting and fun. While the family was busy getting things settled inside the house, the Child was outside playing with an older boy from the new neighborhood.

Why has his subconscious Mind brought us here? I wondered. Each time I reran the event, more detail was revealed. "Feeling good and happy

---

[43] The Wizard of Oz

when everything is new and exciting" soon became "there's too much going on." Feeling good was "too much" for the Child. At first the feeling seemed strange. The Child didn't know how he felt. This was a new feeling! Then, he became aware of a nervous feeling in his tummy.

As he focused on this nervous feeling, he realized that what he was actually feeling was scared, frightened. His subconscious mind was showing us that he was learning that "new" means "threatening."

Once the fear was released, the truth was revealed. The older boy had sexually assaulted the Child. The Child's family was nearby but was unaware that he was in distress. As a result, he had to deal with the experience alone. There was physical pain, intense emotions including terror, and self-blame. Even though, following this traumatic experience, the Child ran to Mum and reported what had happened to him, the initial shock of what had happened to him locked the trauma up inside.

Confession is good for the soul. Here, I use the exact words the Child used, "Pee-pee up my bum." To diffuse the emotional charge, I had him tap while repeating this phrase, again and again. As the client released on this, his body got *very* hot. Fear turned to hate. The more he said the words, "pee-pee up my bum," the more emotion it brought up. Each release generated more heat – a sign of healing.

Releasing the hate allowed anger to come to the surface. Then, shame. Shame is a thought that says, "There's something wrong with me. I'm broken, flawed, worthless."

Releasing the thoughts and feelings associated with shame resulted in a new realization. The client said, "Even though it happened, it's still not my fault." Then, a deeper insight bubbled up, "It's safe to try new things. It's safe to say yes, even though I had this experience. I'm still here. I made it through. I'm okay." It was then that the client was able to find some good in having been through the experience.

Not all things are necessarily "good," but the client recognized that his instincts were good and that he could trust them. They hadn't let him down. His body would never lie to him. This meant that it was okay to trust people because he could trust himself. With this realization, the underlying pattern emerged. "Everything starts out fun and great," he said. "And then I get hurt." He began to recognize how this belief had been formed and then generalized, over time, into every area of his life including personal relationships and finances. For example, "If I fall in love and trust, I'll get hurt."

The client's own "good" feelings had become the trigger. If he started to feel good, his subconscious mind would say, "Uh-oh!" and dump the client back into the emotional chaos associated with the ISE. As a result, he would end up sabotaging his own success. Unconsciously, he had been stuck in an emotional Groundhog Day[44], reliving the pain of the past, over and over, again.

Not a Quick Fix

I saw this client for a total of 16 sessions. Like a snake, he shed layer after layer of false perceptions, painful feelings, and limiting beliefs. When we were done, the client was washed clean of the grimy feelings. Once the blocks from the past were cleared, his mind was wide open to a whole new world of possibility. New information and learning

---

[44] Movie about a cynical television weatherman covering the annual Groundhog Day event in Punxsutawney, Pennsylvania, who becomes trapped in a time loop, forcing him to relive February 2nd repeatedly

were now available to him. I suggested that he give himself permission to finally acquire the knowledge and life skills he needed to create the life he truly desires. And that's what he did.

After a year of personal development studies, he admitted that all areas of his life were steadily improving, including the previous disaster areas of relationship and finances. He was also adamant that, had he not done the regression work, first, he would not have been able to apply himself to the demanding work of self-change.

Solutions that come from the subconscious level of mind are acceptable suggestions. When it comes from the client, this isn't just something you are telling them. You're not just reading them a script. You're feeding back the wisdom of their innermost self. That's potent stuff! Plus, suggestions that come from within are more "brain sticky." These are the client's own truths. If it's a negative suggestion, obviously that needs to change. If it's a positive suggestion, that's gold! Gather these insights and positive suggestions during a session because this is the stuff of powerful direct suggestions. Echo them back to the client at every opportunity. If you deliver them as suggestions before emerging your client, they'll go in like a hot knife through butter.

~ **Dream Healing Practitioner Guidebook**: *A Healer's Guide to Uncovering the Secret Messages of Your Dreams*

CHAPTER 13: SPIRITUAL ISSUE?

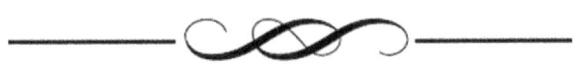

*S*piritual Emergence calls for an appropriate vessel. The ancient healers recognized that, before one can access higher states, there is a need to purify oneself. Unresolved negative perceptions will only contaminate the process. ~
The Devil's Therapy

Some clients will present with spiritual issues that also respond well to regression hypnosis. Spiritual issues can include things like Past Life Regression, Spirit Attachment, Earth Bound Spirits (EBS), Dark Force Entities (DFE) and Extra-Terrestrials (ET). Whether you believe in these things or not, clients will bring them into the session with them. Regardless of what a client's subconscious mind throws at you, to be successful, resolving these sorts of issues requires that you be flexible and adapt to the needs of each client.

Client goes to a Past Life?
Past Life Regression can be useful for discovering hidden talents or finding purpose in this life, but when it comes to solving a specific problem, it can be unnecessarily time-consuming. Whether or not you believe in Past Lives is irrelevant. Many of your clients will. Some will even come to you expecting to go there. The problem is that whatever

the mind *expects* tends to be realized. If your client is a metaphysical type, include a brief discussion about Past Lives in your educational pre-talk to remove the expectation that regression means past lives.

The concept of Past Lives is based on the belief in reincarnation. The basic premise of reincarnation is that we live many lives, and that each life presents the soul with the opportunity to learn and grow. Whatever wasn't learned/resolved in a previous life gets carried over into the next life where it can continue to be worked on as a life lesson. This means that, if an issue has been carried over from a Past Life into the client's present life, so, too, has the opportunity to resolve that issue. This conceptual framework can be used to provide wonderful evidence of the benevolent nature of a Universe which gives us unlimited do-overs.

Even when a client doesn't believe in Past Lives, their mind may go there. Wherever the client goes, that's where you go to work. Just keep in mind the subconscious mind's Prime Directive. Sometimes, it will dive into a Past Life trip as a clever way of by-passing traumatic events in childhood. It could simply be protecting the client from information it deems threatening by avoiding the painful truth of events in *this* life. However, whatever the client's subconscious mind shows you will be relevant to the client's present life and healing.

Whether real or imagined, the event is still coming out of the contents of the client's own mind. The subconscious mind uses a symbolic language that is created through personal associations and interpretations of actual events. Even though the story it shows you may not be factually true, the meaning and emotion trapped in the event is real and can provide valuable information that is relevant to the client's healing. Pay close attention to patterns!

Because the subconscious mind makes no distinction between real and imagined, transforming a metaphoric story can yield real and lasting results. Similarly, exploring a Past Life experience can bring insight into the client's presenting issue. For example, treating a Past Life event "as if" it was the ISE can be a potent contributor to freeing the client from the presenting problem. It can provide some meaningful context for understanding the current life patterns, dysfunctional relationships, and false beliefs. And because the subconscious mind naturally generalizes all change, discharging negative energy associated with a Past Life can weaken or even dissolve events that occurred in *this* life, including the ISE.

Process the Past Life Event
When it comes to therapeutic hypnosis, the standard protocol for processing a Past Life is not much different from working with a current life event. Help the client associate fully into their Past Life Personality (PLP), uncover "what's happening", who's there, and the associated thoughts and feelings, release the blocks, and find forgiveness. Then, find some virtue in the Past Life Personality that can be carried forward into the client's present life. For example, knowledge, gifts, talents, wisdom, positive tendencies, etc. which can benefit the client in their daily life.

Crossing Over Scene
Once the event has been cleared, gather up what was learned from the process and bring it forward with the client to *just before* they are ready to "cross-over" from that (past) life. Pause there, momentarily, to identify the circumstances surrounding the last day of that life. Ask, "Looking back on that life, do you have any regrets . . . or have you come to peace with this life that you are about to move on from?"

Regrets?

Releasing regrets or remorse opens the door for Forgiveness Work. There may have been some sadness about leaving loved ones. Perhaps, there were things left unsaid. This is the time to correct that.

Release any thoughts or feelings associated with dying. If the client's PLP feared for the well-being of their children because of their moving on from that life, guide the client to come to peace. For example, if the client's PLP died of old age surrounded by family, bring awareness to the fact that there was love present. Love heals and they can take it with them.

Violent death?

If that life ended with a violent death, the feelings associated with that end may still be being held onto energetically. As the client releases the thoughts and feelings associated with a painful outcome in a Past Life, peace and well-being are restored to them now. These changes can then be transferred into the client's current life to achieve a lasting result.

Watch your time.

Once the death scene has been processed, instruct the client to, "Relax, let go, and tell me what happens as you leave the body. What's happening?" When the PLP leaves the body, you need to find out if they go into the Light. Watch your session time because, once you move into the between-life space[45], everything typically slows to a snail's pace. This makes the uncovering process very tedious and time-consuming.

---

[45] a.k.a. "inter-life"

A way to speed up the crossing-over process is to instruct the client to "look around and find the light." Suggest that "the Light always comes when a person crosses-over." Then, wait for the client to find it.

Once the client has found the light, give the instruction to, "Reach out and touch the light. Notice how it feels. What's that like?" If it feels warm, loving, and good, the client has effectively moved into the light. You can then deliver suggestions to encourage healing, assistance from loved ones or spiritual guides, and anything else that fits for the client before moving them forward to "just before this life as (Client's name)."

Return to current timeline.
Once you have moved the client to a point just before this life, position the client above their timeline in this life. This is the pre-conception moment which is the perfect place and time to set up for "this life". Treat it as you would the ISE by preparing the client for what life is going to be like. What do they need to know to be able to get through it? Is there something they're meant to learn from those experiences?

How you facilitate the uncovering process will depend on the client's responses, but a tremendous amount of healing can happen in this moment prior to entering their current timeline. Milk it! What's it like in this place? Are they alone or with someone? If there's someone with them, who might that be? Often, clients will be surprised to find they have a spirit guide or a group of angelic beings. These are internal resources that can be utilized throughout the healing process. Just don't try to "install" them. Let it come from the client.

Once the client has a sense of the pre-conception moment, invite them to look at the people who will become their parents. Do they choose these people or is there some other process involved? If they chose their parents, for what purpose? Realize this gives you a wonderful opportunity to begin forgiveness work by exploring parental relationships *before* anything "bad" happens!

Are there any significant people in this life that they knew before? If so, why might they be showing up? Will they be sources of support or teachers? How might these people be helpful with respect to the life lesson the client has chosen for this life?

Have them view the moment of conception, then birth. Find out if they were wanted. Realizing they were wanted can come as a surprise for many clients. If the client reports that they were *not* wanted, find out more. Who didn't want the Child and *why*? For example, maybe Dad didn't want a child and Mom got pregnant. As a result, Mom felt stressed-out. This is an opportunity to reframe the situation. Perhaps it's not that Dad didn't want *them (*after all, how could he? He didn't know them.) But perhaps it's just that he wasn't *ready* to be a father!

Do you see how much healing can happen before the client steps into an event in childhood? Can you see how much easier the forgiveness process will be if you drain off the fears and misconceptions of the child before anything "bad" happens? This is how you can transform a Past Life experience into a current life healing process.

Client Case: The Karmic Wheel[46]

Ellen bounced back to a Past Life where, as her PLP, she experienced a violent death on the battlefield. Her PLP felt remorse for his

---

[46] This session occurred long before I had learned the power of releasing feelings. Had I known then what I know now, I would have done things differently. However, this example illustrates how life-long patterns can be brought to light through a Past Life or metaphoric journey.

misdeeds and his dying thoughts expressed a strong desire to make amends. As the PLP left his body, he drifted up, saw the Light, but did not go into it. Instead, he described a great wheel which he leaped into.

This dropped the client into her next life as a woman in the 1920's. After being betrayed by her boyfriend, she committed suicide. As she was leaving her body, she regretted her decision to take her own life. Then, once again, instead of going into the light, she dived straight into the great wheel, this time dropping into her current life.

The Problem.
What this regression revealed to the client was a theme of betrayal which had been carried over into her present life. She also realized that she was a human soul who hadn't had enough time to process and heal between lives. Desperation drove her to cut corners. By diving into the wheel, instead of entering the light, she skipped past the spiritual de-briefing and healing process available between lives. Each subsequent life only served to reinforce the unresolved emotional pain and feelings of despair. As a result, she grew increasingly more frustrated, remorseful, and self-destructive.

The Solution.
The solution was remarkably simple - identify what's missing and find a way to provide it. We returned to review the first past life and treated it as if it was the ISE. Forgiveness Therapy released the remorse carried forward from that memory. The lessons to be learned in that life were recognized, accepted, and internalized by her PLP before crossing-over. As he left his body, the PLP was instructed to, "Pause for a moment, look back, and find the good in that life." Once the lesson was learned, the PLP was instructed to find the Light, reach out, and touch it.

When a client connects to the light, they are connected to love. It might be the Love of the Universe, or the love of loved ones, but the client can feel it when they reach out and touch the Light. Take advantage of every opportunity to pour in suggestions to amplify "that feeling" because love heals. Fill the client with appropriate suggestions. Then, give them a moment of silence to "soak up all the changes" with instructions to let you know when it feels complete. For example, "Feel the Love. It feels so good. Allowing the Light/Love of the Universe to come into you now, washing, and cleansing, and rinsing, and healing every part of you now – physically, mentally, emotionally, and spiritually. Allowing all connections to that previous life to be released and removed, cleansed, and healed by the Light/Love of the Universe. Releasing and letting go, now, setting you free from the past. Should anything remain, any residual from that life, you can let it go now. Allowing every Part of you to be washed, and cleansed, and rinsed, and healed by the Love of the Universe. Feel it. Know that it's true. Allow it to become a part of you now."

When the client indicated that the process was complete, I said, "That's right. Know that you are loved. Now, take a moment to send *your* love and gratitude to the light. What's that like?" Anything you can do to encourage the client to feel the love will amplify the feeling. It's a yummy experience. If you're short on time, you can use direct suggestions. If you have more time, or want to encourage a deeper healing, use auto-suggestion.

When the client experiences some insight, validate it by having the client say it out loud. For example: "I've changed. I know I've changed because now I feel (put and ending on it) / So now I feel (put an ending on it) / I choose to keep these changes / I take these changes with me – *throughout all time and space*."

Pre-Conception.

Once the client reported that the process of sending and receiving love felt complete, we moved to just a few moments before coming into her present life, bringing all the newer, better awareness' and positive changes with her. This positioned the client immediately before anything "bad" had happened in her current life, allowing us to process this moment *as if* it was an ISE. I instructed the client to look down from wherever she was in that moment, and to look down *into* the life she was about to enter, and from this wiser, more expanded perspective, to tell me what she noticed.

Ellen experienced a profound awareness that what lay ahead in her current life wasn't going to be good. This brought to light negative thoughts and feelings regarding her upcoming (present) life in general. Releasing feelings of apprehension about what lay ahead, and reluctance to "going there" prepared Ellen to face her present life from a place of clarity and empowerment.

Her focus was then directed toward the people who would be her parents in this life. "Notice how you feel toward them as a couple, as well as individually. Did you choose these people to be your parents and, if so, for what purpose?"

Ellen realized that she had chosen a life that would include early childhood sexual abuse, an emotionally abusive mother and, later in life, relationship problems and drug addiction. With clarity, however, she was able to examine her choices and expectations in her current life as a Coming Event. This effectively "pre-pave" the path forward.

Time spent in the pre-conception phase can be rich with insight. Finding purpose in life is like the 'Get Out of Jail Free' card by allowing pre-forgiveness to occur.

If the client is a more spiritual type, encourage them to explore their Pre-Conception Contract with significant people who will appear on their path.

Inform the Inner Child.

Once the client had viewed her current life from the point of view of preparing to enter this life, I had her focus on the little Child that she would become and asked, "As you focus on the little one, still inside Mom, how far along is the Child? Days, weeks, or months?"[47] Then, "True or false - the Child is aware of you and can hear you."

If the client says "false," ask "What needs to happen for the Child to be able to hear you?" Then, invite the client to create that change by telling the Child whatever she wished she had known back then.

As you can see, this mirrors the work you would normally do prior to an ISE. This is a valid opportunity to prepare the Child for the event that is about to occur. In this case, the event is the client's entire life. As this moment in time is long before birth, the Child has yet to experience what it's like to be hurt, or scared, or angry, or feel bad in any way. As a result, you can transform the client's timeline by installing realistic expectations about what lies ahead.

Merge with Child.

Once the client had informed the Child about what to expect from life growing up, I invited the client's spiritual consciousness to merge with the Child. Then, move to just before birth.

---

[47] If you ask how far along the Child is when they join, most clients will tell you that they come and go for the first several months. It seems that the permanent move into the developing present life occurs around 5 months in utero.

Because birth is inherently traumatic, releasing anything associated with the birthing experience can have a dramatic effect on the client's life. Remember, you're setting the client up to be able to cope with how it's going to be growing up *without* having to be overwhelmed or diminished by events in daily life.

Once the birthing experience is clear, you can bring in the adult consciousness of the client to be present at the birth and receive the Child. The goal here is for the client to accept the Child, express love to the Child, celebrate the Child's arrival into the world, and rejoice in the fact that she was finally here, having "made it through." Then, have the client promise to be there for the Child, from now on. From this point forward, it's 'business as usual.' Simply grow the Child up, "bringing all the insights, and learnings, and this newer, better, more expanded level of clarity, peace, well-being, strength, wisdom, etc. forward in time."

As you grow the Child up through the SSEs, test each event, release any residual blocks, and validate the new state of clarity and peace, as you work your way back to the present moment. When the client reaches adulthood, integrate all changes into the present moment – physically, mentally, emotionally and spiritually. Then, send all the changes forward into the future.

Dark Force Entity[48]

Extreme repression of guilt/shame can take the form of malicious entities. These entities have one purpose - to harm the client and effectively destroy any possibility of personal or spiritual growth.

---

[48] An excellent resource for dealing with this issue is Spirit Releasement Therapy: A Technique Manual by William Baldwin and Edith Fiore.

Recognize that these malicious entities are unloved, rejected Parts of the client with roots in the family system. Your preliminary intake should provide clues as to the underlying cause of the problem. Clients who present with these kinds of self-punishing programs always have a religious upbringing. You can read an example of one such case in **The Devil's Therapy**: *Hypnosis Practitioner's Essential Guide to Effective Regression Hypnotherapy.*

A Case of Spirit Attachment

Lisa complained of a pain between her shoulder blades. As she focused on the physical pain, she described it as a dark, heavy, black tar stuck to her back. When she found the emotion that was associated with that "heavy, black tar," it provided a Bridge to the past.

Lisa stepped into her five-year old self, in hospital, having just had her appendix removed. Little Lisa was in a corridor where she found a little girl, about two years of age, wandering the halls. When the toddler told Lisa that she was feeling alone and afraid, Lisa offered to look after the little girl.

Adult Lisa immediately realized that the child wandering the halls of the hospital was dead. In offering to look after her, Lisa had taken on a Spiritual Attachment. This, she realized, was the cause of the "heavy black tar" feeling on her back. Releasing the attachment proved to be surprisingly easy. Lisa simply had a conversation with the dead little girl to explain that carrying her energy was hurting Lisa. As the dead child was not malevolent, she did not wish to cause any harm to Lisa. Lisa reassured the dead child that she was there to help. She then informed the child that there was a place that she could go where she would never be alone, and always feel safe and loved.

At first, the little girl was clingy. She was reluctant to let go of Lisa. But when Lisa said, "Look up and tell me what you notice," the child was awe-struck. "Beautiful!" she exclaimed in wonder.

The suggestion was then given, "When a person dies, the Light always comes. And when the Light comes, someone who knew and loved you will come to carry you into the light. Who comes to carry you into the beautiful Light?"

Once the Child recognized the loved-one who came with the Light, she felt safe in reaching out. The moment she touched the hand of the loved one, she crossed-over into the Light. Following this session, Lisa's back issue cleared up.

All Parts formed to meet important needs for safety, nourishment, and comfort. Every Part deserves to be treated with kindness and respect. Even angry or malicious Parts. Problem-causing Parts are often a problem because they have been judged and rejected. Angry, destructive Parts are often Child Parts that have been deeply wounded and need to be loved and accepted in order to heal.

~ **The Devil's Therapy**: *Hypnosis Practitioner's Essential Guide to Effective Regression Hypnotherapy*

CHAPTER 14:
GOT FORGIVENESS?

F*orgiveness is not something that we do. It's something that happens when you let go of negative emotions. Release everything unlike love and you won't have to convince the client to do anything. The forgiveness will happen automatically. To accomplish this, the client must be willing to release all the anger toward the Offender.* ~ **The Devil's Therapy**

Forgiveness is a letting-go. It is literally the moment the client lets go of *the problem*. If you're looking for the holy grail of healing work, this is it. Releasing internal stress restores a person's ability to relax physically. Stress inhibits cognition. Releasing results in greater mental clarity which opens the door to insight and greater understanding. Understanding is the threshold of forgiveness.

Everything in the therapeutic process has been leading up to this. Authentic forgiveness restores a person's sense of safety in the world by restoring their power of choice. As a result, they feel like they're back in control of their life. When forgiveness is authentic and complete, there's simply nothing there to generate any of the symptoms. That's the goal of regression hypnotherapy - lasting change. But don't push for forgiveness. When the client is ready to love and accept herself. When she's ready to let go of the petty stuff (and it's all petty stuff) forgiveness will happen effortlessly.

Like most things, the ideal setting for the forgiveness work depends on where you're at in the process. For example, forgiveness of the Inner Child can take place at the ISE. As the client forgives their younger self, they are forgiving a Part of themselves. This makes the client stronger.

Often, the root of the problem is the Child's inability to accurately interpret what was happening during the ISE. If no real crime was committed in the ISE, once the Child has been restored to feeling safe and secure, you can invite Grownup to, first, forgive the Child. Then, forgive any Players in that event. Later, when you conduct the forgiveness work toward the main Offender, you can test and then compound any forgiveness that has already been established.

The Steps:

1. Forgive the Child.
2. Grow the Child up.
3. Integrate changes.
4. Forgive everyone who showed up in the regression.

Step 1: Forgive the Child.

The root of all negative emotions is fear. Clearing the ISE means releasing the fears and misperceptions of the *Child*. Once you have released those fears, the client will be able to think clearly, perhaps for the first time. This is the opportunity to generate some incredible insights!

Before growing the Child up, ask the client, "What have you discovered? How does this change things?"

CH: Knowing what you now know (offer a mini review of what the client has learned) is there *anything* you could have done to change things? After all, you were only two years-old!"

Recognizing that the Child couldn't have done anything to change the event makes the Child forgivable. If the client is still blaming the Child, the ISE is not clear. Remember, the Child is a Part of the client. Blaming the Child is anger towards *self* which is calling for correction.

When the client answers correctly by saying, "No" (there's nothing Child could have done), follow up by suggesting, "Then there's nothing *wrong* with TWO, is there." Notice that this is a suggestion - not a question.

Client: "No!"

CH: "That's right! She just happened to be there, right? Nothing personal." (Children personalize *everything*. We want to "unplug" this. Remember, if there's nothing wrong with the Child, then there's nothing wrong with the client. They simply had an experience.)

Client: "That's right!"

CH: "Bring your attention to that beautiful little Child. Isn't she lovely? And so brave, too! Isn't that true?" (Make the Child a hero!)

Client: "Yes."

CH: "Can you accept her – just as she is?" (Acceptance of a Part is an act of self-acceptance.)

Client: "Yes."

CH: "TELL HER. Say, 'I accept you – just as you are.'"

Client: Repeats – using autosuggestion.

CH: "Does she believe you?" (Test the acceptability of the suggestion)

If the Child *doesn't* believe Grownup, say, "Inside of you are the words TWO needs to hear so that she *can* believe you." (Let the client do the work!)

If the Child *does* believe Grownup, say, "She believes you! You've changed! Look at that precious little one . . . If you had a little one like her, a little daughter or niece . . . could you *love* her?"

> Never introduce love until you've tested for acceptability. Love equals acceptance but we want to introduce the concept of self-love gradually. This ends the internal battle.

If the client says, "Yes" instruct her to *tell* the Child, "I love and accept you just as you are. You are precious to me. (Fill the Child with love, acceptance, appreciation, etc.)" Then, have the client notice how it feels. It should feel good.

If it feels good, have the client repeat the words and notice how much *better* it feels. (i.e., use autosuggestion to compound the suggestions) Then, follow up with the whammy, "Even though TWO has done nothing wrong . . . do you *forgive* her?"

Grownup will typically say, "There's nothing to forgive." To which you reply, "That's right. Even though there's nothing to forgive, *tell her.* I love you. I accept you. I forgive you. Even though you've done nothing wrong, you're loveable. You're good. You're forgivable, etc."

As you can see, this is pre-paving the way to self-forgiveness. All forgiveness is self-forgiveness. By the time you get to the final step of the healing process, most of the forgiveness work should have already occurred. All that's left to do is test and verify the forgiveness that has been accomplished, and release whatever is left.

Step 2: Grow the Child up.

Regression hypnotherapy is a process of self-discovery. To release the underlying cause of the client's presenting issue, you need to identify (a) how the seeds of that issue got planted in the ISE, (b) how that problem grew and developed over time through the SSEs, and (c) how these events eventually found expression as symptoms.

How did the seeds get planted? As the client releases the painful emotions trapped in the ISE, the client will experience greater mental clarity and self-awareness. You can take advantage of this natural process by asking questions to elicit insight. For example, "What are you discovering? What's changed?"

While insight isn't necessary to resolve the client's issue, it can sure speed up the process. All you need to do is gather up all the insights and better feelings, established in the ISE, and invite the Child to "grow up" to the next SSE knowing what she now knows, feeling good about herself, and filled with resources which now empower her.

Transforming how the ISE feels will often change the SSEs because, had the block never formed in the first place, this is how things would have played out. i.e., the Child would have made it through the ISE without a loss of security or self-worth.

Grow the Child up through the SSEs knowing only love and acceptance. This will allow you to test to ensure that all blocks revealed in the ISE have been completely neutralized. This, then, reinforces the "truth" that change has, indeed, occurred. It also allows you to uncover any subsequent issues that might have been added to the overall problem.

Step 3: Integrate changes.
The Child embodies the changes that occurred at the ISE and was reinforced through the SSEs. These changes need to be delivered to the adult client.

Integrate all changes at adult level of consciousness. Positive changes which have occurred need to be transferred to the grownup level of awareness. Bring all insights, wisdom gained, and feelings of empowerment forward from the ISE to the client in the here-and-now. This prepares your client for the final step in the process we call Forgiveness Work.

Step 4: Forgive everyone.
Unforgiven Parts represent unresolved grievances. As such, they have the power to continue to generate unwanted symptoms. Remember, the people who were responsible for harming the client in the past have been internalized as Parts. Understand that when the client forgives these people, he is forgiving himself. All forgiveness is self-forgiveness.

When it comes time to forgive a Perpetrator of harm, you have options. You can either create a scene or guide the client into a familiar place.

In either case, it should be a place where the client can feel safe being themselves.

Gerry Kein's Grey Room is ideal as a created scene for forgiveness work. If you want to amplify the emotion of anger, make the color of the room red.

If the Offender is a parent, ask the client where they would like to meet with this person. For example, the kitchen table is a familiar place that has association with the parent at the age they were wounded.

If the Offender is no longer alive, take the client to the deceased's graveside. Then invite the client to get it out. Make it safe for the client to release the hurt, fear, anger and guilt. Start by spitting on the grave. This can give some perverse pleasure while acting as a warmup for speaking the words that need to be said.

If the Offender is a deceased loved-one, you can take the client to the deathbed scene. Regardless of how the loved-one died the client can still experience the relief that comes from taking care of old business. Saying those final words can be very cathartic.

Other options include a special place like a garden or the seashore where they can be visited by that person. This is more of a bereavement technique, but even when the client insists that there is nothing to forgive, there is always anger for things said or done, and there is often reticence to express that anger. Providing the client with an opportunity to say the things they didn't get to say while the person was still alive can bring closure and peace.

Before facing the Offender, remind the client that the Child is innocent, didn't know any better, couldn't have done anything to change what happened but *they can*. The Child is blameless. There's nothing wrong with the Child. The Child didn't have the problem, Offender has the problem. Then, direct the blame toward the Offender. This will bring up the anger toward "that person."

The key to healing is to allow the Truth to be spoken. Letting the client know that "they" won't remember anything once the conversation ends can dissolve inhibitions.

Troubleshooting Forgiving the Child

Nothing really "bad" happened?
If no real harm occurred, i.e. the event was just misinterpreted by the Child, go for the forgiveness. Say to Grownup, "Focus your attention on (Mom) and notice how you feel *now* . . ."

Forgiveness is an *effect* of releasing fear, blame and anger. If the blame and anger has been released, forgiveness has already occurred. Because the emotional charge has been neutralized, the client will feel only love toward Mom. This is when you can formalize the forgiveness by having the client look at Mom and say, "I forgive you Mom. I set you free. Even though you did nothing wrong . . . I forgive you. As I forgive you, I set *myself* free."

Bad things happened?
If something really bad happened, there's nothing we can do to change that. Any attempt to change the event will only generate internal dissonance. The solution is to guide the client to accept what happened, then convert that level of acceptance into self-acceptance.

For example, autosuggestion statements might include:

- It happened.
- I made it through.
- I survived, I'm still here!
- I'm stronger now.
- I'm not a Child, anymore.
- I've changed.
- I'm not that person anymore.
- I've learned from that experience. (positive learning)
- What has been learned can be unlearned. (negative learning)
- I can choose to heal.
- I can choose to forgive and set myself free.
- I'm allowed . . .

Child took the blame?

Trauma survivors take the blame for the things that happened to them as children. This needs to be corrected because a person cannot feel good about themselves in a state of shame/blame/guilt/resentment toward self or others.

The Child needs to be forgiven by Grownup for not-knowing, not being braver, giving up, doing or not-doing, and all the perceived "shoulds." For example, "Even though (specific perception) it's not your fault. You were just a child. You didn't deserve it. (*You're* not the problem – Mom has the problem.) And even though *it happened*, you're allowed to grow up feeling good about yourself because no one knows you better than I do. I'm *you*, all grown up, and I love and accept you, just as you are. You're good enough. You're smart enough. You're capable enough. You're allowed to grow up knowing that and feeling that way, too. You're everything you need to be to (tie to therapeutic goal) because I love and accept you. And even though you've done nothing wrong, I forgive you."

800-pound gorilla in the room?
Some clients grew up in an environment of abuse. Some have survived horrific events which left them traumatized. If there's a person who harmed the Child, e.g., molester, the Child doesn't need to forgive that person. The Child only needs to release the fear generated by that experience and be brought to the realization that the event is over.

Forgiveness Work requires adult consciousness. Children are naturally forgiving. They forgive, over and over, again. It's by doing so that they can survive a childhood of abuse. But, over time, the subconscious mind can turn the person who hurt the Child, i.e., Offender, into an 800-pound gorilla. That gorilla is the accumulated anger being carried by the adult client. This needs to be purged by the *adult*, not the Child. Standing up to the "monster" who hurt them as a Child will instill a much-needed sense of power.

Troubleshooting Growing the Child Up

New aspects in SSE?
If you uncover aspects in an SSE *which were not in the ISE*, resolving them is usually simply a matter of reframing their significance. However, some issues can have multiple ISEs. If the aspect does not yield to surface techniques, conduct the ISE test for "that feeling." i.e., "New or familiar?" Regardless of the client's answer, Bridge back to the "first time."

SSE tests clear?
When the SSE tests clear, use it to generate more insight by inviting the (older) Child to think back to the ISE when he had "that problem."

You can then take a moment to celebrate how the Child has changed, is changing, and will continue to grow and change as result of what he now knows. The Child is learning and, as a result, growing wiser and stronger. Point this out! This encourages the client to look forward to more positive change as they "grow up" through the SSEs.

Troubleshooting the Testing and Integrating

Is the ISE completely clear?
Can the client move through the original event, just as it happened the first time, without getting triggered? Can they move through the event as an observer, feeling calm and relaxed? Can they get through the event feeling good about themselves?

Has everyone been forgiven?
Is the client still blaming the Child? Remember, the Child is a Part of them that needs to be forgiven. What specific grievance is the client still holding onto? The answer may be the key to their healing!

When they mentally picture the Offender, do they feel peaceful? If they experience even the slightest twinge of fear or anger, release it. Remember, saying the words, "I forgive you" is a test. Does it feel true?

Is there someone you missed?
Even a person who was *thought* of during the ISE needs to be forgiven. Remember, forgiveness is a letting-go. If someone comes to mind during an event, the client needs to let go of any guilt, shame, blame or unrealistic expectations associated with this person.

Troubleshooting for Complete Forgiveness

Is the ISE completely clear?
Can the client move through the original event, just as it happened the first time, without getting triggered? Can they move through the event as an observer, feeling calm and relaxed? Can they get through the event feeling good about themselves?

Has everyone been forgiven?
Is the client still blaming the Child? Remember, the Child is a Part of them that needs to be forgiven. What specific grievance is the client still holding onto? The answer may be the key to their healing!

When they mentally picture the Offender, do they feel peaceful? If they experience even the slightest twinge of fear or anger, release it. Remember, saying the words, "I forgive you" is a test. Does it feel true?

Is there someone you missed?
Even a person who was *thought* of during the ISE needs to be forgiven. Remember, forgiveness is a letting-go. If someone comes to mind during an event, the client needs to let go of any guilt, shame, blame or unrealistic expectations associated with this person.

Resistance to facing Offender?
If the client is reticent to face the perpetrator, remind her, "You're not a child, anymore. It's your turn to take back your power and speak the truth. Do that and it ends right here and now. This is where your miracle lies. You get that out and you're free!"

Resistance to expressing anger?

If the client is avoiding their anger or starts making excuses for the perpetrator, review the facts. For example, "True or false, he hurt you when you were just a little girl?" Then, invite the client to tell the Offender (a) what he did, (b) how it impacted her as a child, (c) how it continues to negatively affect her through symptoms. For example, "Tell him – you hurt me! You stole my innocence! You made me think I was worthless! You put all this fear and anger inside of me!"

Build up the emotional charge. Then, guide the client to find the words and pump the feeling into the pillow.

An empowering technique is to name the pain and then give it back to the Offender. For example, "I give you back your hurt! I give you back your fear! I give you back your anger! I give you back your worthlessness! I do whatever it takes. I don't carry you inside me anymore. I give you back all your pain.'"

When the client has exhausted the emotional charge, invite her to take back what was taken from her. For example, "I take back my innocence. I take back my right to feel safe. I take back my worth. I take back my ability to love and be loved."

Forgiving a Parent?

Once the client forgives a parent, say to the Parent, "There's probably some things you need to forgive (Client) for." Inviting the Parent Part to forgive the client can remove hidden guilt issues which color the client's relationship with their parent.

Partial forgiveness?

Remember, forgiveness is a by-product of the releasing work. It's not something we do. It's something that happens when we consciously decide to stop holding onto the pain of the past.

If the client is still holding onto some of the pain, they still have the problem. But you won't know if you don't test. Is the anger gone? Is it *all* gone?

If the client reports partial forgiveness, take a SUD. How much is still left? Remind the client that the goal is 100% forgiveness because that's 100% freedom. If they only forgive 50%, it's like leaving a little infection in the wound. They'll feel better for a while, but only 100% will give them a lasting result.

How old is the client? If the client is advanced in age, partial forgiveness may be sufficient to carry them through until they expire. If they're younger, it's only a matter of time before they experience a recurrence of symptoms.

Forgiveness requires Adult Consciousness because forgiveness is about releasing anger. The Adult (CM) is carrying the burden of unresolved grievances while the Child carries the fear. Is something in the client's past still calling for resolution? If so, find the thought/feeling combo that has everything to do with "that anger." Follow it back to the vent that caused it. Once resolved, come back to the forgiveness process. Much easier.

Toxic relationship or home environment?

If the client's home life is toxic, reluctance to release the anger is understandable. Remember, anger is about protecting boundaries.

You can replace the protective mechanism of anger with forgiveness. For example, "Forgiveness will release you from bondage to the past. Not only that. Your forgiveness will protect you from hurt, from negative words someone might throw at you. If someone were to throw hurtful words at you, it might *seem* like arrows coming at you, but those arrows will just fall away. Or maybe they just bounce off you, like you're coated with Teflon, or surrounded by a lovingly luminous light. Whatever they throw at you, it's like water off a duck's back. This is because, when you forgive, there's nothing negative on the *inside*, so it just can't stick. In fact, if someone were to throw hurtful words at you - some negativity or criticism - the more they throw at you, the stronger you feel that calm serenity inside of you."

Forgiveness actually feels good. During the Ready for Regression Session, you have the ideal opportunity to show the client that there's no reason for fear. It's just that forgiveness is not what they think. Forgiveness based solely in reason is just head forgiveness. That's what most people think forgiveness is. The problem is that the heart is screaming out to be heard. And until somebody has the heart to listen, the mind and body will continue to suffer.

~ Tribe of Healers: Ready for Regression First Session Course

CHAPTER 15: UNFORGIVEABLE?

*W**hen the client can look upon the Offender and see them as forgivable, their own self-concept changes. Remember, the Offender is an Internal Representation of how the Child perceived the Offender in the ISE. What's hurting the client now is holding onto past grievances in the form of anger, resentment, blame, and condemnation. This is a self-punishment program. The client has been punishing himself, in the privacy of his own mind, by holding onto the pain of the past. Worse, all the unresolved toxic emotional debris from the past has been contaminating the client's present life and all their relationships. And because they have internalized the people who hurt them, until they forgive, they will continue to suffer the symptoms.* ~ **The Devil's Therapy**

When a client is unwilling to forgive because the person who hurt her "doesn't deserve to be forgiven", realize the client is not yet convinced that forgiveness is the right thing to do. Take a step back and continue to educate the client about the cost of unforgiveness and the rewards of letting go of the pain of the past. Begin by saying, "You're probably right. What they did to you was wrong. But here's the thing . . . Your forgiveness isn't for them - it's for you." Then, remind the client that keeping herself in prison because of what the Offender did doesn't hurt "that person" - the only person it hurts is Client. Offer the reassurance that the Offender doesn't have to *know* that they have been forgiven because forgiveness is not for them. Client doesn't have to tell them, or have contact with them, or be nice to them. Forgiveness isn't for them – it's for Client – so that she can be free of the symptoms. i.e., free to heal.

Offender is perceived as "evil"?

If the Offender is unforgiveable because the client views them as "evil", you can use the Windows of the Soul Technique[49] to make the offender forgivable.

Windows of the Soul Technique

First, establish that every "evildoer" was once an infant. Then, as every infant is innocent, something must have happened to Offender to change that. Then say, "It's been said that the eyes are the windows of the soul. What this means is that, when you look into a person's eyes, you can see all the way back in their time - all the way back to when they were just a tiny baby – when all they wanted or needed was to love and know that they were loved. Look into those eyes, now, and tell me what you see.

"As you look at that tiny, little baby, it's as if you can see through his eyes. Look inside Mom and notice – something's off. Inside of her are all her unresolved grievances, pain, hurt, and anger. Perhaps, already you're beginning to realize how *desperate* she must have been . . . for love. And how *burdened* she was by her *own* unmet needs, fears, and inadequacies. She put those things inside that innocent little baby. "She wasn't *able* to gaze into the eyes of her *own child* and see him for how he was. She didn't see a beautiful human soul, did she? She didn't

---

[49] Gerald Kein Windows of the Soul Technique

recognize that a precious gift had been delivered into her care. How could she? She couldn't see past her own hurt and pain, could she?

"Do any of those things have to do with the child?" (The child is just there, isn't that true?)

"How does this affect how Mom views the child?"

"Does she love and accept the child, or something else?"

"Does she *want* to love the child? But can't?"

"What about Dad? What problems are in him?"

"Notice all *his* grievances, *his* pain and hurt and anger. Do those things have anything to do with the child?" (The child is just there.)

"How do the unmet needs in Dad influence how he views the child?"

"Notice the child taking it all in without the benefit of critical thinking. Notice the confusion, fear, and hurt, because of those things. What is the Child learning?"

"Journey forward over the first three years of his life, and notice how it is to be this child, with these parents, in this family, culture, religion, etc. What is the Child learning about how to be and not be?"

"What is the child being told?"

"What is being modeled to the child about (relationship)?"

"What words or behaviors are being taken in and shaping his identity?"

"What expectations are being placed on the child?"

"Notice all the pain, and hurt, and anger *because* of those things. What are you discovering?"

"Journey further ahead and discover what it's like to be growing up in this family. In childhood, what caused him to lose his innocence?"

"At what point does the child turn "bad"?"

"In his teens, who did he have to become to survive?"

"Did he feel confident, kind, self-assured and secure? Or insecure, striking out in a battle to survive?"

"As a young adult, was it safe for him to trust? Or did he have to close his heart to others?"

"Now see him as a grown man. How must he feel inside to be able to act in such unloving ways?"

"The seeds of the adult are in the child. The seeds of wounds that were perpetrated on *you* are in *that child* who was neglected, or mistreated, or abused. It was at the hands of another that he grew to act out in hurtful ways. And it was coming out of the pain he was carrying inside. You see that now, don't you?"

"I wonder . . . how far back might that wound go? How many generations before it found its way to you?" (Optional: Intergenerational Timeline)

"We're not here to make excuses, only to understand that this was a wounded soul striking out because of all the fear, and anger, and guilt trapped inside. That pain was put there by *others*. You know how that feels. (This suggestion generates compassion.)

"So, now you have walked a mile in another man's shoes. Can you see how *that child* didn't have a choice? The child was a *victim*. The consequences, unfortunately, impacted *you*. But it wasn't personal. That goes back lonnnnnng before you were even conceived" (This suggestion heals betrayal.)

Intergenerational Timeline

"Researchers have discovered that trauma gets passed on generationally. For example, anxiety can be passed down through generations. The sins of the fathers *are* visited upon the next generation as cellular memory. But this does not need to be a prison sentence.

"The whole idea of Karma is that it's your kettle of fish. What you do with it is up to you. The burden is also the gift. The challenge is one of finding the gifts in the garbage because, what you most need to learn, undo, and overcome in this life is what you will teach, or demonstrate, or give to others."

Instruct the client to go back *before* the pattern ever existed, before the energy was created. This may go back many generations, but the objective is to go *before* the pattern was formed. This is the ISE – an inter-generational causal event. It is very easy to remove the pattern once the client lands at its inception because, like a past life regression, there's an element of dissociation and the characters are complete strangers.

Review from above the timeline and do the uncovering process as an observer. Then, drop down into the timeline *before* the causal moment. Do the clearing there.

Test that it's clear. Then, send that new energy forward along the ancestral timeline so that all future generation may be healed. (Native Americans say we have a responsibility to heal our ancestors. That's what we're doing – healing the ancestral lineage through a timeline generalization process.)

Send the energy all the way up to the birth of the Perpetrator. (The client is bestowing a gift on the person who hurt them.) Test that the child has received this new energy/information. Then ask, "How does this change things for the child?"

Send the energy forward along his timeline. "How does this change things growing up?"

Send the energy into the moment where Offender's path intersects with the client's path. How might things have played out differently with this truth? (This is a mental rehearsal of the wished-for past so let the client fulfill that need. What you find is the victimization of the client doesn't happen. Subconsciously, the client is learning that nothing happened. That's the forgiveness.)

Bring that transformational energy up to the client in the present moment. The client will be able to look the Offender in the mind's eye and feel only the love. Then say, "*Even though* that's not how it happened, looking back at that moment your paths crossed, if you had known *then* what you know *now*, you might not have ever achieved this depth and breadth of healing.

"Understand this wasn't just for you. You are healing many generations of wounded souls. This is no small thing. The ripple effect goes out into the Universe. It affects everyone. Take a moment to accept the Love of the Universe. Feel the gratitude. (continue blathering to compound the good feelings)

Bringing Down the Wall Process

If the Offender is a loved-one - for example, a parent or a sibling – realize that the client has, out of necessity, erected a protective barrier between themselves and the person who hurt them. That wall needs to come down. This will allow love to flow back into the client, transforming every aspect of their life including all their relationships.

The Steps:

1. Autosuggestion process.
2. Forgiveness warmup.
3. Establish a contract.
4. Dialogue process.
5. Wrap up.
6. Set up for more forgiveness.

Step 1: Autosuggestion process.
"You know that we're having these sessions because *you are determined* to overcome this problem. It has controlled your life long enough. You are determined to *take charge* to set yourself free. Your subconscious mind understands that, now, and realizes that *you are ready* to get that problem resolved now and forever. You're allowed to be happy. You're allowed to set yourself free from the past and move on. It's simply a matter of motivation.

"You've punished yourself long enough (and you know that's true.) And even though you might have changed this pattern sooner - *had you known how* - it is now time to forgive and rewrite history. Ready?

"Here's how we'll do it. Make a soft fist and place it gently over the region in the center of your chest. That's right.

In a moment, I'm going to say some sentences. I want you to say these sentences with me and, as you do, gently rotate your fist in a clockwise direction. Understand?

"Say these sentences strongly, but silently, *in your mind* with me. As you do, *feel* them. *Believe* them. *Make them real* with an honesty and enthusiasm that now make these words your truth. Okay?

"All right. Take a nice deep breath, hold it, and as you exhale relax and go deeper. Very good.

"Even though I might have blocks to forgiving / I deeply and completely love and accept myself.

"Even though it's sometimes hard to forgive / I deeply and completely love and accept myself.

"Even though I have created patterns of struggle and pain and suffering / I deeply and completely love and accept myself.

"I'm ready and grateful for this healing. / I'm willing to forgive and set myself free.

"I'm now willing to forgive everyone / in my past or present / living or dead / who has ever hurt me in any way.

"I am now willing to forgive anyone and anything / that has contributed to (problem) / and the part they played.

"I am now willing to forgive completely / and set them free / to set *myself* free completely.

"Even though there may be other blocks / that I don't even know about / I deeply and completely love and accept myself.

"And I am now ready to forgive *myself* / for any hurt I may have caused others / either knowingly or unknowingly / understanding I did the best I knew how in those situations / and I'm changing.

"I now choose to use those events / only as learning experiences / to help me do better in future.

"I am now willing to forgive my parents. / They did the best *they* knew how.

"I am now willing to forgive *myself*/ for not changing this pattern sooner. / It is now time.

"I am now ready, willing, and able / to forgive everyone and anything / that might have contributed to me having (problem.)

Step 2: Forgiveness warmup.
"Now, take three deep breaths and, as you do, experience the power of forgiveness coming into you. With every inbreath, *feel* your connection to this power, the power to release, to let it all go, and set yourself free. With every exhale, let go. Let it all go, once and for all, and make room for a new energy, a new frequency of change. That's good.

"Now, take a moment to imagine someone you truly love and have a warm feeling toward. Someone who is not a parent. It might be a special friend or a sibling or a child. Who comes to mind?

"Notice how that feels – the warmth, the connection, the love that's there. Where do you feel that? (Inviting the client to describe it will amplify the feeling.)

"Stay focused on that feeling while I have a talk with your subconscious mind. Subconscious, I'd like you to review the history of this (special) person. Do a search for any scenes, situations, or events where they might have said or done something hurtful to (Client). Any situation where they might have stood in (Client's) way, or caused them pain, or derailed them. Whatever they did or failed to do – at the snap of my finger, Subconscious, show the consequences of these events.

"(Client), let your own mind show you the effects of these things, and what feelings you feel, as the subconscious mind surfaces those incidents and grievances. 1, 2, 3 (snap!)

"What feelings? (Heaviness in chest? Gut? Head?)

"So, now you have a sense of how, no matter how you might have set it aside, or tried to disguise your true feelings, those feelings are still there. Realize those feelings have been keeping a wall between you and (person) so that when you're in the same room as that person, or even hear their name, those unwanted feelings are still present. Whether they're right out front or buried just beneath the surface, those feelings are there, even though you *want* to be loving toward that person.

"How do you suppose it would feel to just bring down that wall that's been between you? Would you experience more love? More laughter? Would you be more forgiving toward one another? That's why we're here. (Goal statement) by returning to love."

Step 3: Establish a contract.

"In a moment, I'm going to ask you three questions. I don't want you to *think* the answer to each question, I want you to *feel* the answer by simply pausing just long enough to allow the question to sink down to that deeper part of your being where your true feelings will make themselves known to you.

"You may feel different feelings – that's good. Feelings are natural and have probably been there for quite a while. Just let them be there and give yourself permission to experience them.

"The answer to these questions is either "yes" or "no." Any other answer such as "maybe", or "I think so", or "I'll try", or any other vague or qualifying answer, counts as a "no." Qualifications don't come from the heart. They come from the head. Understand?

The first question is, "Would you be willing to forgive this person *totally*. By this I mean, are you willing to let go of everything that's come between you, and release the guilt and fear, by not keeping any part of it for later? Because that's what it means to forgive a person totally. It means you are willing to no longer be bound to them in this way.

"We're not making excuses for them. Just the willingness to say, "I no longer take it personally. I just learn and move on." And to come from that place of wisdom that understands that everything we do is literally dictated by our subconscious mind – so they couldn't have behaved in any other way. That's just how it was.

So, let yourself feel the answer now. Would you be willing to forgive this person *totally* - "Yes" or "no"?

The second question is, "Are you willing to forgive this person *absolutely*? By this I mean, are you willing to give up your favorite stories and scenarios about them – the things you say, again and again, about how they are, and how that affected you? (pause) Because these stories and scenarios have had a lot of juice for you in the past, enough to *keep* you in the past. Are you willing to release the past, give up permission to use those stories, either with yourself or with others? Because that's what it means to forgive a person absolutely. It means you're willing to permanently erase that bit of personal history that's contributed to your book of emotional scars. It takes a lot of heart and courage to forgive another, absolutely.

So, let yourself feel the answer now. Are you willing to forgive this person *absolutely* - "yes" or "no"?

The third question is, "Are you willing to forgive this person *unconditionally*? By this I mean, are you willing to give up permission to entertain characterizations of them. A characterization is an image of a person we create in our own mind. It has nothing to do with the person. It only has to do with what you *think* about them. Are you willing to give up those characterizations – not just now, but forevermore - even though they may do what they usually do, which has upset you in the past?

"From this moment on, giving up permission to use what they say or do to form characterizations of them, recognizing that it really has nothing to do with this person. It only has to do with what you think about them. So, once again, would you be willing to forgive this person *unconditionally* - "yes" or "no"?

Step 4: Dialogue process.

"Now, the fact that you have brought *this* person to sit in front of you says that you are willing for *some* forgiveness to take place between the two of you. Your heart is open to them, right now, and there may be something you want to tell them from your heart. (pause)

"So, right now, I'd like you to open your heart and let it speak through your throat, and through your mouth, in whatever words you need. And tell them everything that's there for you to say, *as if you may never see them again.* (wait)

"Now, there may be some things they want to tell you from *their* heart. Some gratitude, perhaps, or something they need to forgive *you* for. (Switch to the other person and wait)

(Continue dialogue process until client comes to peace.)

"That's good. Just let that be complete now. And in your mind's eye, I want you to look deep into that person's eyes. Become aware of what you see. What do you become aware of?"

"Do you forgive them totally? (Yes) Nothing personal, right?

"Do you forgive them absolutely? (Yes) So, the past is just the past, right?

"Do you forgive them unconditionally? (Yes) Realize, they haven't changed. *You* have changed – so you can heal. Understand?

"Say it, "I have changed / I know I have changed because (put an ending on it.)

Step 5: Wrap up.
"There is a moment in time when all things wrong can be made right. That moment has been called the holy instant. It's a sacred moment that exists outside of time. The instant a grievance is released, *healing* flows in to replace it. You've experienced that sacred moment, and now you know what it really means to forgive. What did you discover?

"Feel peaceful? Let yourself smile inwardly as you sink down deeper into that feeling of peace because you have learned something very important here today, something that very few people ever get to realize. Tell me – is forgiveness worth having?

"Now that you know what it means to forgive, you realize that you've been punishing yourself by holding onto grievances, right?

"You've been depriving yourself of the gifts of forgiveness (go through the benefits of resolving the presenting issue).

"What might your life be like in the absence of *all* those grievances? What new decision for your life would you like to make because of having had this experience?

"From this day forward, every decision is going to become very simple because every choice either leads to happiness, or away from it. As we continue the work together, realize there will never be a problem in motivation again. *Now you know* what forgiveness can do for you. And you want all your choices to be for happiness, isn't that true?

Step 6: Set up for more forgiveness.
"Would you like to experience more forgiveness? (Yes.) Thats good because even more forgiveness will release even more of the guilt, and fear, and hurt, and condemnation in *your own mind*, that's been making

your mind a living hell. Forgive everyone and everything – then you're free. And you realize it's not saying that what another did or said was okay, but only to understand that they just couldn't figure out how else to do it. They couldn't figure out how to overcome the inner programming that caused them to act in unloving ways, right?

"Forgiveness does not condone an act. Forgiveness is a willingness to just drop your expectations of them and say, "I let you be human, I let you be whatever you need to be. I no longer expect anything else." That's what allows *you* to be free – and to be at peace!"

What Forgiveness is NOT

1. Forgiveness is NOT condoning what was done to hurt you.
2. Forgiveness is NOT excusing bad behavior.
3. Forgiveness is NOT denying what happened.
4. Forgiveness is NOT minimizing the hurt.
5. Forgiveness is NOT forgetting what happened.
6. Forgiveness is NOT religion.
7. Forgiveness is NOT telling the person you forgave them.
8. Forgiveness is NOT reconciling with the Offender.
9. Forgiveness is NOT giving up having feelings.
10. Forgiveness is NOT merely words.

Sources:
Gerald Kein, Omni-Hypnosis
Cal Banyan, 5-PATH
Fred Luskin, Forgive for Good
Beverly Flannigan, Forgiving Yourself

CHAPTER 16: THE CORRIDOR METHOD

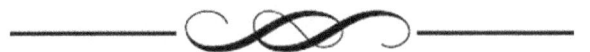

The uncovering procedure makes the unconscious conscious. As a result, there's always going to be some resistance to allowing the details to come to full awareness. The conscious mind will naturally want to question the process. Don't let that happen. Keep the focus on the feeling. The feeling is the key that opens the door to the event. ~ **The Devil's Therapy**

The Corridor Method is a versatile imagery exercise that you can use as a regression technique, or as a preliminary diagnostic/uncovering technique. The structure of this technique lends itself easily to a shorter session because not all doors need to be finished during one session. When one door is completed, the next one can be addressed in the following session.

Once you have established a state of hypnosis, instruct the client to imagine a set of stairs leading to a deeper level of awareness. Then, use a deepening count as you guide the client down to this deeper level. Suggest that, when the client reaches the count of one, she will find herself in a corridor where she will find whatever you want the client to find. At the count of one instruct the client to step into the corridor and notice the doors on either side of the corridor.

Preliminary Uncovering Technique

If you're using the Corridor Method as a preliminary diagnostic or uncovering technique, you can give the suggestion that behind one of these doors lies the answers or the resources needed by the client. Then, give the suggestion that the door will make itself known to her. It will stand out, in some way. For example, it may be a different color or shape, or Client may just sense or feel that this is the right door.

When she finds the door, invite the client to describe it to you. This is a subconscious symbol that can speak volumes about what the client is discovering! Find out how it feels to be standing on this threshold. If necessary, provide safety. Then, be prepared! Invite the client to open the door and step inside. What do they discover?

Regression Technique

If you're using the Corridor Method as a regression technique, give the suggestion that the further down the corridor the client goes, the further back in time she travels. Each door can be blank, or it can have a number on it signifying the year or the age of the client.

The Corridor of Forgiveness

This variation on the Corridor Method is a direct approach to dealing with guilt by introducing a path to self-forgiveness. You can use this process to uncover the people and situations which the client is refusing to face and forgive.

As you'll see, you can easily blend this process with other techniques. For example, regress to cause, bringing down the wall, higher states, etc.

The final stage in the process is designed to formalize forgiveness of self. You can also utilize this process following the standard forgiveness protocol or as a stand-alone process to generate further insights.

The Steps:

1. Stairway deepener.
2. Establish the Corridor.
3. Make forgiveness reasonable.
4. Find the door.
5. Describe the door.
6. Explore what's behind the door.
7. Gain a higher perspective.
8. Cancel guilt thoughts.
9. Return responsibility.
10. Integrate.
11. Make permanent.

Step 1: Stairway deepener.

"Find yourself at the top of a stairway leading down to a much deeper level of awareness... down to the storehouse of your mind where old accounts are kept, and campaigns are decided.

"In a moment, I'm going to count from ten down to one. As I do, feel yourself moving on down that stairway. At the count of one, you will find yourself at a much deeper level of awareness. 10, 9, 8, 7, 6, 5, 4, 3, 2, and ONE."

Step 2: Establish the Corridor.

"We're now at the bottom of the stairs. Find yourself in a corridor that sweeps out in front of you. This is the Corridor of Forgiveness. At the end of the corridor is another set of stairs leading to the final Door of Forgiveness through which *you* will be completely forgiven. Then you'll be free. But before you can enter the final Door of Forgiveness, there are other doors, doors on either side of the hallway, through which you can forgive the past. Behind each door you will find some scene, situation, or person that, once forgiven, will allow you to enter the Door of Forgiveness and be released from the symptoms.

"When you have fully forgiven, then there's nothing there to support the problem. As you forgive, you heal. And I don't know how much you *need* to forgive, but I do know that there's an ancient wisdom that says, "do unto others as you would have done unto you." Whatever we do to another, we do to ourselves in our mind. That means that, as we forgive, we *undo* what we've been doing to ourselves. *Then* the Door of Forgiveness will open to us."

Step 3: Make forgiveness reasonable.
"Before we begin, it's important that you remember what it means to *be forgiven*. It means you're going to be better. When you enter through the Door of Forgiveness you will be transported into a very special place, a spiritual place for many, a place of peace, and joy, of unimaginable love. But to get to this place, where you can *know* what it means to be completely forgiven, it is necessary to release the past. You *do* this by forgiving everyone and everything that ever hurt you. Only then will you truly be *ready* to be forgiven.

"You'll be free because, in your mind, it will be as if nothing ever happened. This is not to say that those events or situations didn't occur. Forgiveness doesn't change the past. It changes how you *feel* about the past. You remember it in a new way. And when you have forgiven completely, your forgiveness will expand into the future with new, positive possibilities because the mind is no longer a place of condemnation. Perhaps you're already beginning to realize that it costs you nothing except pain, bitterness, guilt, anger, and all the negative thoughts and emotional energies that have been keeping you in (symptoms) hell.

"Forgiveness is your Get-Out-of Hell-Card because those events, while they might not have been what you would have preferred - and some were challenging at the time - it is still possible to find some good in them, some strength or wisdom to benefit you by making you healthier, wealthier, wiser, happier, and more complete.

What "good" might that be - I don't know. *You* don't know. But your *subconscious* mind knows, and you can discover this for yourself, and find your peace - a marvelous state of invulnerability - that easily enables you to overcome this and any problem."

Step 4: Find the door.
"In a moment, we're going to begin moving down the corridor. And your subconscious mind can direct you in a way that easily enables you to forgive in a way that allows you to develop increasing strength and skill by forgiving.

"Realize that the Part of you that has inner wisdom, or is most closely connected to God, or Universal Mind, or Holy Spirit, would never give you an assignment without first ensuring that *you have the resources* you need to succeed completely. So, your subconscious mind can begin with those people or situations that are *easiest* for you to forgive, and as you come to understand the information from a more *mature* point of view than you had when the information went into your mind, you'll gather more resources and *learn* how to release the problem completely.

"As you look down that hallway, you may get a sense of which door you would like to enter first. A certain door will stand out to you - as if there's something special about this particular door - indicating that this is the door through which you can forgive today and move that much closer to the inner purity of your true self.

"And I don't know how many doors we need to pass through before you realize *complete* healing, and *total* freedom, but I know that your mind is receiving guidance and is enabling you to be released from the problem.

"Now, begin moving down the corridor, and when you have found that door, I'd like you to describe the door to me, even the doorknob."

As the client moves down the corridor, continue building the energy of what it means to forgive.

Step 5: Describe the door.
When the client finds the door, begin the uncovering procedure by inviting them to describe the door to you. Take note! The subconscious mind uses symbolic language. Is it an old door? This might suggest that behind it lies an event from the past. Is it a prison door? This might suggest ongoing entrapment and punishment within the mind!

Don't rush the process. Give the client time to build the image. For example, "What do you notice about this door? What color is it? What sort of material is it made of – wood, stone, metal, or something else? How does it open - with a doorknob, a handle, or something else?"

Dial into the feelings associated with the door. For example, "What told you that this is the right door? Does it feel like it's new or familiar? How does it feel to be standing on the threshold of this door?"

Invite the client to reach out and grasp the handle or doorknob and notice how they feel. Remember, their subconscious mind knows what's on the other side of the door. Apprehension could be a precursor to an abreaction! For example, "As we stand here together, reach down, and grasp the handle, and notice how you feel. In a moment, I'm going to ask you to go ahead and open that door and tell me what's inside. What feeling are you feeling?"

Step 6: Explore what's behind the door.
Invite the client to step inside. Treat the scene as you would an event in a regression session. You might just get a spontaneous regression. Yay!

Build the image and emotions associated with the scene. Gently tease out the information. For example, what's the client's first impression as they step inside the room? Does this place feel new or familiar? What time of the day might it be – daytime or nighttime? Are they alone or is there someone with them? Who? What are they noticing? What's happening and how does that make them think or feel?

If the client steps into an empty room, that's resistance. Clearly there is something the client is trying to avoid. Say, "Well, maybe there's an adjoining room. Let's see if we can find it." Then invite the client to seek and find the hidden entry-point to the scene that is calling for healing.

If the room is dark, there's something the client doesn't want to look at. What feeling are they feeling? What would make them feel better?

Let the client find their own solution. For example, would bringing more light into the situation be helpful? If so, invite the client to find something - a light switch, flashlight, lantern, or some other method of bringing light into the room.

If the client is resistant to seeing what's there, give them control over how much is revealed at once. For example, install a dimmer switch then turn up the lights in increments. Releasing trapped emotions will decrease resistance to allow more awareness of what's happening in the scene.

When the scene has been fully explored, understood, and/or neutralized, exit the room, and return to the corridor. Have the client close the door behind her to symbolize completion. i.e., leaving something behind, as a memory.

If you have time, find the next door that calls to the client. Otherwise, wrap things up for the next session by having the client return to the stairway. Then, return up the stairs with an emerging count.

Step 7: Gain a higher perspective.
Following the forgiveness process, guide the client to follow the corridor to the end where they will find a stairway or elevator leading upwards to a higher level of consciousness. You can use an increasing count with intermittent suggestions of rising upward and feeling lighter and lighter.

Once the client arrives at the higher level, you can invite the client to connect with their higher self and, from this higher perspective, view their issue, receive guidance, insight, and forgiveness. Be creative! If the client is not spiritual, take them to a higher vista where they can look over their entire life and see all the benefits of having forgiven those people. Invite them to connect with their internal source of guidance. Who comes? Alternately, you can suggest their Wise Mind[50], Future Self, Guardian Angel or someone who has crossed over to the other side who loves them. For example, "Sense or feel that Part of you that has protected you, loved you, and nurtured you all the days of your life.

Invite the client to "feel the compassion and love, acceptance, wisdom, dignity, peace, and forgiveness radiating from them and flowing into you, now." Then suggest, "It's all in you now - that deep knowing of what is best for everyone concerned and with it the ability to see the whole sweep of history, how all things are connected, all people past, present, and future.

From this perspective, you can look back at your personal self, and all the Parts that comprise the whole personality, and all its history, background, connections, and future possibilities. So, from this vantage point, you can see how life is such an interesting learning ground, and how you were a person experiencing life and learning through it.

"And as you look down upon that timeline, whatever you did in the past, whatever you might do in the future, is looked upon with the wisdom, the patience, the love, and forgiveness, and deep knowing that there's nothing wrong with you. There never was, never will be.

"And you realize, sure, you've made mistakes. We all do – that's how human beings learn. Human beings were created to grow and develop and learn through trial and error. We do that best in love and

---

[50] Marilyn Gordon, The Wise Mind: The Brillian Key to Life Transformation and Healing

understanding. No mistake could ever negate, in any way, the presence of your (higher self), and the love that's there, that understands that mistakes are steppingstones to wisdom.

"As you can look down upon your timeline, you can see yourself more completely, with all your history, every event, every feeling, every triumph, every mistake, every lesson, and the skills you have developed to date, and you can look upon it all with more love, isn't that true?

"And perhaps a deeper appreciation for what you are *capable* of becoming because there's so much *experience* there, so much wisdom now. And as you look at the world through new eyes, and see things so differently, realize there is no greater hell than guilt, is there? Guilt demands punishment. You realize that now, don't you?

"And how some people choose to punish themselves by depriving themselves – of adventures, perhaps, or privileges, or by holding themselves back in some way. Some deprive themselves of relationships that would enhance their lives if they'd let them. Or by depressing themselves and putting down their positive qualities. Some even go so far as to convince themselves that they have no right to live. They feel so unworthy that they tell themselves they don't deserve health, happiness, life, even. So, as you look at the world, you bring it all together into a new understanding for yourself, a new wisdom that will enrich *your* life."

Step 8: Cancel guilt thoughts.

Ask the clients (higher self) to release and replace guilt-based thoughts and the uncomfortable symptoms they generate. For example,

- "Are there any beliefs that can now be released and replaced?
- "What are they?

- "Are there any beliefs that have caused Client to punish herself, or deprive herself, in the past?
- "Does Client have permission from (higher self) to cancel these old beliefs and all the effects?
- What new beliefs can now replace the old beliefs in a way that restores Client's capacity to freely forgive and remain free?

Instruct the (higher self) to cancel the false beliefs and replace them as a permanent part of the Client. Then test to make sure that the process is complete. For example, ask the client's (higher self):

- "Have all false beliefs about Client been cancelled? Does Client believe this?
- "Have the guilt or bad feelings about X been cancelled?
- "Has the belief that Client doesn't deserve to live a long and happy life been cancelled?
- "Does Client understand now how the events in the past caused the problem?
- "Have any negative tendencies that have contributed to the problem been cancelled? Now and forever? Does Client accept this?
- "How does this change things from now on?
- "Is there anything else Client needs to know and hear at this time? What counsel can (higher self) now offer?

If the process is not yet complete, what needs to happen to make it complete?

Step 9: Return responsibility.
The (higher self) knows everything about us including everything we have ever done, thought, and said. Because the (higher self) is the

source of all healing, this Part of the client knows their true purpose for living. Why not ask it! For example, "Client, are you now willing to find a new purpose for living – a purpose aligned with your (higher self)?"

If the client says, "yes", switch to (higher self) and say, "I'd like you to now return responsibility to Client for the way she leads her life, okay? And you'll be sending your love now, without conditions, to nurture Client on her path, right? Okay, go ahead and tell her in whatever words she needs to hear."

Then, test. Does Client accept it? Is she willing to take responsibility from now on? If not, ask (higher self) to come up with a solution to this obstacle.

Step 10: Integrate change.
"Client, I'd like you now to just experience your Higher Self taking these new resources, insights, and capacities that you have just created for yourself into the rest of your past, into every experience that needs to be re-evaluated and released in the same way. Give your wholehearted permission for your (higher self) to do this, now.

"Imagine it radiating the power of these new resources, seeking out and re-evaluating all these experiences *in light of your purpose for living*, and transforming them now in the same way, into resources for you, as new learnings, and new affirmations of your inner purity, and inner strength, and capacity to take care of yourself appropriately, now."

What's that like? What is the client discovering? What else?

This is the gold! Milk it!

Step 10: Make permanent.

"Now, there's just one last thing. Client, are you now willing to keep this change within you *intact*? In other words, are you willing to commit to vigilantly keeping this wisdom and learning by using it in your everyday life in an ongoing way?

"You do that by *remembering*, first, how to avoid similar errors and, second, how to think, feel, and act more lovingly, wisely, and with more inner strength, instead of the old patterns. Are you willing to keep this change *intact*?"

If the client says, "Yes", instruct her to say it out loud. "I will keep this change in me intact." Then say, "And so it is, *not because I say so*, but according to your will. Nothing could ever take away your free will. Say it again, "I *will* keep this change in me intact!"

If the client says, "No", ask (higher self) to identify the block and come up with a solution.

Step 11: Wrap up.

Thank the client's (higher self) and all Parts for doing such an awesome job. Then say, "The process is now complete. Forgiveness is complete. You found your peace. That means you're not the same person anymore – *are you*?"

"You've changed. And because you've changed, your future is now bright. Your commitment to keep this new pattern intact ensures complete and total restoration of health, happiness, peace, and well-being, to all your systems.

"Naturally, things are going to continue to occur in your life, and sometimes things happen that may not match our preferences. That's life! You realize that now, don't you?

"*No matter what*, you stay committed to keep this new pattern, right? You hold onto the love. We're not here to try to change the world. We're here to set you free by removing any expectations that the world be anything other than what it is – and still be okay.

"In future, any regrets or disappointments will be short-lived, at best, and much easier to process and release quickly. In this way, you remain free."

Continue to reinforce change during the post-emerging debriefing. For example, "You've done some powerful work here today. You realize that don't you?

"Repeat this sentence and put an ending on it"

1. The learning for me in all this has been . . .
2. I know I've changed because . . .
3. I will keep this change intact because . . ."

High frequency level work expends a great deal of mental energy. As a result, tiredness later is common. This is because the body is resting and playing catch-up while the mind is working very hard to integrate all the changes. A simple homework assignment to support integration can be very helpful. For example, "You might want to do some journaling over the next several days. And to reinforce all the positive energies, create a drawing to represent these powerful changes and place it where you can see it."

Post-Forgiveness Healing Patter

"Let yourself go deeper down now, deeper inside, deep inside your heart now, and let my words flow over you like a warm and gentle rain. Imagine above you a beam of golden-white energy flowing down into the top of your head. A beautiful, radiant beam of healing light coming down from the heart of Creation. And it bathes and rinses every part of you.

"Feel that beautiful golden, radiant white light moving down your body, around each arm, and around each leg, surrounding you with its loving energies, saturating every muscle, fiber, gland, organ, tendon, bone, nerve, cell – every aspect of you, body, mind, and soul.

"Your soul drinks thirstily from the golden white healing light as it comes down from the heart of Creation. This light of Creation goes down into your heart. The *love* of Creation goes into your heart, your heart filling with the energy of love, and gratitude, and appreciation for the beauty of forgiveness, the blessing of letting forgiveness be done *through* you.

"Well-being now streaming powerfully through your entire being, washing away anything that might have stood between you and complete healing. Every fiber of your being, down to the atom, is radiant with the power of forgiveness to heal your life and bind all things together in perfect harmony.

"Your DNA is transformed as the love of Creation streams through you, every part of you welcoming it, drinking it in, filling you with the peace and strength and the confidence that allows you to just let it stream out into the world, now, bringing peace to every mind. That's what your forgiveness can do.

"What's that like?"

"Hold onto that feeling and realize it lets you move about freely. It's invisible to anyone else but you can feel it, the strength it brings you, the protection."

Self-Forgiveness Practice

An effective self-healing practice in forgiveness is Ho'opono'pono, as taught by Dr. Hu Len[51]. This is something you can do on your own and teach to clients as a clean-up routine following a session. In general, you can use it as an autosuggestion technique, but if a stronger emotion gets triggered, combine it with tapping to get a deeper release.

First, when an uncomfortable feeling gets triggered, don't think. You don't need to analyze what just happened. Just make the decision to release it using the following sequence:

1. Focus on crown chakra and say, "**I love you**." For a spiritual client, have them say this to their Higher Power.

2. Focus on brow chakra and say, "**I'm sorry**." You don't need to know what you're sorry for. Just recognize that an uncomfortable feeling has been triggered and you are willing to let it go.

3. Focus on heart chakra and say, "**Please forgive me**." Remember, forgiveness is a giving up of *the problem*. You're giving it over to a higher power, whatever you imagine that to be.

---

[51] Zero Limits: The Secret Hawaiian System for Wealth, Health, Peace, and More, by Joe Vitale and Ihaleakala Hew Len, Ph.d.

4. Finish with, "**Thank you**." This is a statement of trust that the triggered aspect has been removed. While there may be other related aspects that will need to be removed, "that feeling" does not need to be re-experienced.

This practice can be done anywhere in the privacy of your own mind. Simply say the statement silently to yourself. To increase focus, add tapping or place your hands over each of the chakra points. Finish with open hands, i.e., open to receive forgiveness.

The signature of the ISE is what I call the SEAL Pattern. This is an acronym that defines the four aspects that you really need to watch for when you're doing the uncovering work. SEAL stands for:

***S**hock*
***E**motional Intensity*
***A**lone*
***L**ack*

~ **Tribe of Healers Root Cause Remedy for Results Course**

CHAPTER 17: LASTING RESULT?

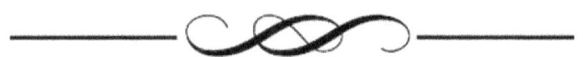

Think of the time between sessions as a soaking in period where suggestions for change will either take effect or be challenged. If nothing changes, nothing changes. So, something should happen between sessions. The client may feel better, worse, or experience some ups and downs. This provides the information you need to guide the healing process effectively. So long as something is happening between sessions, progress is being made and tells you what needs to happen next. ~ **The Devil's Therapy**

During a regression session, your client will typically revisit some events from childhood. They'll release some emotions, gain clarity, and gather up some resources and better feelings. They'll emerge feeling better than when they arrived in your office. In some cases, the client will float out of your office, feeling transformed. But don't be too quick to pat yourself on the back and think, "What a great job I have done!"

While you can try to convince a client that change has occurred, they won't be truly convinced until they see the evidence for themselves. That's when they will fully appreciate your good work!

If you don't test, you won't know. And if you don't know, you may fail to get a lasting result. It won't be until the client returns for their next session that you'll know whether the results are truly going to last. This is the benefit of scheduling a follow-up session.

The Steps:

With regression hypnotherapy, the four most important tests are:

1. Test for compliance.
2. Test for state.
3. Test for the ISE.
4. Test the results.

Step 1: Test for Compliance
Hypnotherapy requires the client's participation. Is the client following your instructions? If you don't test, you won't know.

Step 2: Test for State
Real regression requires somnambulism. Is the client in a state of somnambulism? If you don't test, you won't know.

Step 3: Test for the ISE
The Initial Sensitizing Event (ISE) is the situation responsible for generating the symptom(s). It's the "first time" the client ever felt "that feeling." A complex issue, with multiple symptoms, can have more than one ISE feeding into it. But you won't know if you don't test the results – both in session and between sessions.

Step 4: Test the Results

While you can use techniques during a session – for example, mental rehearsal or future pacing can be used to test the client's expectations - the only true test of the *results* occurs in the client's daily life.

Change doesn't happen in the session - it happens *after* the session. That's when post hypnotic suggestions take effect. While you might think you did a bang-on job in the first session, you won't know if the problem has been completely resolved, or whether the client can keep the changes, unless you test the results in their daily life.

When your client leaves your office, their subconscious mind is naturally going to continue to work on their issue. As a result, the client may experience additional insights or realizations after the session. Feelings, emotions, or memories may bubble up to the surface. They may even have interesting dreams. All these things are evidence that their subconscious mind is working behind the scenes. The question is, "Can the client hold onto the changes?"

Scheduling a follow-up session will allow you to test the results in the client's daily life. Internal changes will always be reflected in the outer conditions of the client's daily life. This makes the time *between* sessions just as important as the session itself. If there's a problem, the subconscious mind is going to let the client know. This is the information you need to guide the healing process effectively.

You simply cannot override the protective function of the subconscious mind. You must provide evidence to both the conscious and subconscious minds that it's safe to allow change to happen. This is true at every phase of the healing process. For example, we educate our clients about the healing process because you can't make a person heal. They must be willing to participate in the process by following your instructions. You cannot tell a client anything that they do not already accept to be true. The client can, and will, reject any suggestion that goes against their deeply held beliefs. They will hold fast to their subconscious "truths" - even those that are a source of pain.

While you can encourage the subconscious mind to hold onto all changes through the process of integrating and generalizing change[52], the fact remains that when a client leaves your office, they return to their daily life. That is "what's normal." And whatever they consider "normal" acts as a support system for their presenting problem. After all, "normal" is where all the client's triggers hang out and that includes people and situations you know nothing about.

Like it or not, clients don't always tell you everything. If the client withheld some important piece of information, or you overlooked something that turns out to be critical to their healing, or it's something that just didn't come up during the session, that unresolved aspect is going to fester. Leaving something behind is like leaving a little infection in a wound. It's going to fester. This is the leading cause of symptom recurrence, recidivism, and conversion.

If the client experiences a recurrence of symptoms or unwanted behavior, this tells you one thing – you're not done, yet. There is something at a subconscious level of mind still calling for resolution. The good news is that when something happens to trigger a recurrence, that situation/event in daily life can serve as a means of targeting the underlying cause of the problem. Releasing the cause is the way to ensure a lasting result.

---

[52] Remember to keep a record of significant SSEs while you're Bridging back. This will allow you to come back to complete the healing process by testing and compounding all changes as you grow the Child up to adulthood.

Like housework, healing is a process. When a house has been neglected for too many years, you can end up with a big job on your hands. It can take time to accrue sufficient emotional healing to tip the scales in the client's favor. This is essentially what is occurring throughout the healing process - the client is accruing increments of change. Some of these changes will be significant. Others will be quite small. As each increment of change is recognized and accepted, order will gradually be restored to the client's mind.

Order is the antonym to chaos. Chaos is a state of stress, strife, struggle, and pain. That's the problem. As a newer, better level of order is established, the client's mind will become increasingly receptive to suggestions for more empowered ways of thinking, feeling, and behaving. All you need to do is gather up each increment of change and validate it. Then, use these shifts in awareness as *evidence* that positive change is occurring.

Make note of each shift toward the better, then, at the end of each session, deliver it back to the client in the form of direct suggestions. Suggestions based on the client's own experience are statements of truth! As such, these suggestions will make a lasting impression.

Healing is not a race for the finish line. It's a journey of self-discovery. Your work is not done until the client can hold onto the results. Take heart! Even when you haven't completely resolved the client's issue there can be unexpected benefits. Because of the subconscious mind's natural tendency to generalize change, positive changes can be reflected in *other* areas of the client's life before their therapeutic goal has been achieved. Any conscious recognition of change will allow more change to happen.

Preliminary Check-In

The purpose of conducting a preliminary check-in before each session is to identify what needs to happen next in the client's healing program. The check-in gives you a natural way to pick up where you left off. Think of it as a continuation of the previous session. You're simply picking up where you left off.

Begin by inviting the client to do a little mental rewind of the previous session. Then ask, "What do you remember about that session?" Sharing in retrospect will help to step back into the previously visited events, while refreshing your memory, and can provide clues as to what needs to happen next in the client's healing program[53].

What happened?
What happened following the session? If your client was able to hold onto the changes between sessions, great! Whatever you did in the previous session was effective. Something has changed! Celebrate it! Compound any recognized shifts toward the better. Leverage them as evidence that change is occurring. Then, poke around a little. Did you get everything, or is there something else? What's left? Build positive expectancy for a complete resolution of the problem. Then, focus on "that feeling."

If your client was *not* able to hold onto the changes between sessions, great! What happened? As the client reflects on what happened between sessions, watch for a spike of emotion. Is that the *same* feeling that came up in the previous session? Or is it a *different* emotion bubbling up to conscious awareness?

---

[53] You can learn more in Ditch the Script: Set Up to Wrap Up for Successful Regression Hypnotherapy

Sometimes a client will report feeling worse following a session. When this happens, don't take it personally. It's not that you did anything wrong. Hypnotherapy naturally stirs up subconscious content. What you need to find out is – is it the same feeling or a different feeling? And what, if anything, happened to trigger it?

Same feeling?

Did you find the ISE for "that feeling"? Did you clear everything in the ISE? Did the client realize how that experience resulted in the unwanted symptoms? Did you test the results and generalize all changes while growing the Child up? Did you Future Pace to test the client's expectations in future?

Use a directed regression to go back to the event visited in the previous session. Then, conduct a quick review using the basic uncovering questions. What's happening? Who is there? How do these things make the client feel? What thoughts are being generated? How do they make the client feel? Stir up "that feeling" powerfully then Bridge back further. If the client goes to an earlier event, you'll know you didn't have the ISE for "that feeling."

> **Note:** *the feeling is specifically defined by the thought. For example, the thought, "I'm going to die!" and the thought "I'm not wanted" both generate the emotion of fear, but they're not the same fear. Pairing the thought and the feeling together will give you a more targeted Bridge to the ISE.*

If you did, in fact, locate the ISE in the previous session, you probably missed something. Remember, to get a lasting result, you need to clear everything. Then, there's nothing left to generate the symptoms. Titrating the event can help you to isolate the specific thought-feeling-response pattern. Remember, the thought generates the emotion. When you uncover a thought, reality-check it with Grownup by asking, "Is that true?" For example, "Is it true that (Mom doesn't want you)?"

If the thought is true, the uncomfortable feeling is reasonable. For example, if Mom wanted to abort the pregnancy, what does the Child need? How can Grownup satisfy that need?

> **Note:** *the subconscious mind will withhold information that it feels will be too overwhelming for the client. Remind the client that whatever happened, they've already lived through it. They survived. It's just a memory but the subconscious mind doesn't know this, yet. It doesn't know that they're not a Child. As a result, it's still trying to protect them. Then, invite the client to say out loud, "I can handle it. I'm allowed to feel it and I'm allowed to heal it."*

Different Feeling?

When a new feeling comes to the surface of awareness between sessions, this is good news! What probably happened in the previous session is that you poked a hole in a pocket of venom and the subconscious mind has been ruminating on it, ever since. Great! "That feeling" has everything to do with the client's problem. It's a subconscious signal that can lead you right back to the event that caused it, and you don't have to go digging for it. It's right there beneath the surface. This gives you the next step in the client's healing process.

First, remove any doubt by satisfying the conscious mind's need for a reason. The client needs to recognize that whatever happened in the last session worked. This is something new coming to the surface and should be taken as *evidence* that the subconscious mind wants the problem resolved. Clearly it trusts you. As a result, it is pushing all the gunk up the surface where it can be dealt with. Remind the client that "there's only so much of that in there." Second, instruct the client to focus on "that feeling."

If the client is willing to allow the feeling to come up powerfully, you won't even need a formal induction. Remember, the stronger the emotion, the deeper the hypnosis.

Assign Homework

You can use a homework assignment as an overt test of the results between sessions. In this case, the homework assignment serves as a contract the client makes to take a specific action. When a client is willing to participate in their own healing between sessions, the healing can be deeper, and results can be achieved much more quickly. But for the contract to be binding, the client must be ready, willing, and able to act on it.

Clients who are willing to do homework between sessions make better clients because they're more invested in achieving the results. But if there's *any* resistance to doing the homework, it's probably too soon to consider it. When a client is resistant to making a change, it's not their fault. There's a subconscious block preventing them from taking appropriate action. Identify what the specific block is to taking action. It may, in fact, be pointing to a major contributor to the client's presenting issue.

The type of homework you assign should be consciously chosen and effortlessly acted upon. It should support the client's healing process and, ideally, should be an extension of the session-work, based on what has been revealed or cleared in hypnosis.

Homework should never be used as a task/expectation of performance. Assignments that demand performance can sabotage the client's success by undermining their faith in the hypnotherapy. Remember, if the client was able to make those changes on their own, they wouldn't need you.

Before you assign homework, be clear about your purpose for doing so. Homework should be used to:

1. Empower the client.
2. Reinforce positive change.
3. Test the results.

Empower the Client

If your purpose for assigning homework is to empower the client in their daily life, come up with something that the client can easily do. For example, a coping technique such as tapping, or self-hypnosis can help to empower the client between sessions.

During the post-hypnotic interview, when a client has clarity that suggests taking action, challenge the client to come up with one small, specific action they can take that is congruent with this new level of awareness or insight. Then, elicit a verbal agreement from the client to take this action before the next session. When the client acts, based on subconscious information, the subconscious mind learns that the conscious mind can be trusted to listen.

If you can come up with something the client enjoys doing that can support them in achieving their healing goal, they'll be more likely to act on it. For example, many clients enjoy journal writing.

Writing daily can be especially therapeutic and can help to deepen the client's healing. Journaling can bring to light insights and reinforce changes that occurred in session. It can also bring to awareness unresolved aspects or deeper layers which can then be addressed in subsequent sessions.

When the client successfully accomplishes a homework assignment, you can use it as evidence of success. They're doing something to move themselves in the direction of their desired goal. Validate this! Encourage them to feel proud! Even the smallest measure of success can be used as evidence of the client's ability to be successful. This will increase positive mental expectancy and hasten the achievement of the client's therapeutic goal.

If the client is reluctant to take action, it may be that they perceive the task as too daunting. If it feels like it's too much, it probably is. Chunk down. If necessary, reduce it to the ridiculous[54]. For example, if going outside for a 30-minute walk every day feels like too much, how does going for a 15-minute walk every other day feel? If that feels like too much, get creative. How does the client feel about putting on their walking shoes every day?

The key is to be specific. What will the client do? When will they do it? How often will they do it? Get a verbal agreement. Then, keep the client accountable by following up in the next session.

Reinforce Positive Change
If your purpose for assigning homework is to reinforce positive change, it needs to be congruent with what came up during the session. For example, during Future Pacing, you can encourage a weight-loss client to imagine using the Finger Pinch Technique frequently,

---

[54] A really good book on this is One Small Step Can Change Your Life: The Kaisen Way by Robert Maurer

throughout the day, to feel calmer and more in control. The homework assignment is then to use the Finger Pinch frequently throughout the day.

Test the Results

Whatever happens between sessions is just information. It's not a measure of success or failure. If the client fails to follow through with an agreement to do homework, this tells you that there is resistance to allowing that change. The homework assignment then serves as a test. In this case, the homework assignment has successfully brought to light a subconscious block.

This tells you what the next step in the healing process needs to be. Resolving this block will free the client from bondage, allowing them to act in alignment with her consciously held desires.

Secondary Gain

Secondary gain may be a factor if you're working with the conscious mind, but there must be a *primary* gain before there can be a secondary gain. The primary gain is called the Symptom Imperative. The Symptom Imperative is the subconscious mind's purpose for generating the problem in the first place. That's what the client is paying you to bring to resolution.

Symptoms always serve a positive purpose. It's just that the conscious mind doesn't like them. But if you take care of the primary gain, the secondary gain issue will often take care of itself. At the very least, once the underlying subconscious need has been satisfied, it will respond well to surface techniques.

A Case of Intense Anxiety

Leanne had been seeing a psychologist for years to deal with her social anxiety, but he hadn't been able to get her anxiety-driven eating behavior under control. When Leanne's doctor expressed serious concern for her health, she knew that she had to get her eating under control. Diabetes ran in her family and Leanne was dangerously overweight. She knew that her weight problem was a result of her high-level anxiety.

During the intake, I asked Leanne what she thought was the worst contributor to her weight problem. Without hesitation she replied, "Chocolate, and not the good kind, either."

Leanne then revealed that she kept a drawer full of chocolate bars in her bedroom. Her nightly routine was to binge on goodies while watching TV. We then established an initial therapeutic goal which was to get rid of the chocolates - a feat Leanne was certain would be impossible.

We agreed to keep the focus on the emotional release work. The homework assignment – throwing out the candy bars – would serve as a way for us to test the results. When Leanne could throw out the chocolate bars, she'd be back in control of her eating.

As agreed, each session focused solely on releasing feelings. (This was a case of intense anxiety that literally shook the chair.) Each subsequent sessions, Leanne would report back in and each week the score was:

Chocolate Bars - 1

Leanne - 0

While Chocolate continued to hold power over Leanne, she began noticing several interesting side benefits of the releasing work. For example, she noticed that she was feeling good about accepting invitations to Christmas events – something she normally avoided. In fact, she was surprised to find herself enjoying socializing with friends. The goodies in the workplace were still a temptation, but her confidence was beginning to rise. Leanne was experiencing a new sense of control over her choices.

By session 6, Leanne proudly reported that her score board had changed dramatically. She had successfully dumped the contents of the junk-food drawer into a garbage bag and taken it out the curb. Leanne was beaming with pride because Chocolate no longer had the power to control her. This was the turning point for Leanne. It was also her final session with me as she wanted to continue working with her psychologist. Her final session focused on celebrating success. But how successful was she?

Several months later, I was out for a walk around the lake with a friend who brought her dog along. My friend struck up a conversation with another woman who was out walking her dog. This woman started sharing with my friend how amazed she was to be free of her lifelong addiction to chocolate. It was then that I realized it was Leanne! I didn't recognize her because she had lost over fifty pounds!

As this usually socially avoidant woman kept chatting away with a complete stranger, Leanne began to reveal how her newfound freedom had resulted in her ability to finally let go of her house and move into a new apartment. In doing so, she had left behind all the negative associations from her past. More importantly, symbolically, Leanne had moved on into a new way of life.

As you can see, homework can be a highly effective way of testing the results between sessions. Changes that occur in session will automatically be reflected in the client's daily life. When the client fails to act it's not a failure. It's a successful use of a test to uncover the block to the client's ability to take the desired action. When you release the blocks, change will happen very naturally, often in the most surprising ways.

The Tapping Solution

Tapping[55] makes a great homework assignment because it's a releasing technique that you can use in your regression sessions. Once the client has learned how to tap, it can then be assigned as homework. This gives the client a self-healing, self-empowerment technique they can use anytime, anywhere, to feel better.

Tapping makes an effective coping strategy because it's always right at your fingertips. It can be used to support the client between sessions while you continue to work on resolving the overall problem.

Once you're confident that the client knows how to do the tapping sequence, you can suggest it as a homework assignment. Two sessions are usually all it takes to give the client enough hands-on experience working with you to feel confident tapping on their own.

Five minutes practice, once or twice a day, is a good start, but be sure to let the client know that she can use it anytime she feels the need.

---

[55] Also known as Emotional Freedom Techniques or Meridian Tapping Techniques, tapping is an evidence-based approach which belongs to the field of Energy Psychology.

The following general approach to tapping has been adapted from the Tapping Solution by Nick Ortner.

Step 1. Find it.

Go inside and think of everything that's been bugging you. Make a list of every annoyance or upsetting little thing. Be petty! Whatever has been dragging you down, or draining your energy, bring it to mind. Then, put it into a ball.

Step 2. Feel it.

Close your eyes and focus on the ball while tapping. Do several rounds and watch the ball melt away to nothing.

Step 3. Heal it.

When the ball has completely disappeared, tap on all the positive and good things you want in your life. Fill the void with something good.

Step 4. Seal it.

Acknowledge the difference you feel in your mind and body. You just shifted your energy! Good job!

Simple Energy Techniques (SET)

Steve Wells and Dr. David Lake of EFT Downunder have developed their own approach called Simple Energy Techniques (SET). One of the cornerstones of SET is continual tapping. The 'Boys Down-under' suggest that increasing the amount of meridian stimulation is a key factor in the improved results they're seeing. They aim to get as much tapping as possible into every session. I figure why not?

Continual tapping is a great tool for empowering a client and it's something they can use, right away. It's easy to do, it's non-fatiguing, and anyone can do it.

Daily tapping will decrease stress levels and increase positive energy. It seems to have a 'toning' effect on the energy system that can alleviate problems the client may not even be thinking about. There's no need for a set-up statement or even a specific focus. All the client needs to do is tap, rub, or hold any of the points, in any order, until they feel relief.

Covert Tapping

Another easy technique Wells and Lake came up with is tapping or pinching the finger points using the thumb of the same hand. The client can use this technique anytime and anywhere – driving in the car, standing in an elevator, talking on the phone, sitting in a meeting, watching TV, or any stressful situation where they want to experience the calming effects of tapping.

This gives the client a technique they can use, in times of need, without anyone knowing that they're tapping. For example, you can tap when you're in an elevator surrounded by strangers. The worst thing that can happen is someone might think you're keeping time to the muzak.

Covert tapping is discreet, so doing it in public won't draw unwanted attention. And it puts relief right at the client's fingertips. Simply tap on or pinch the finger points on the hand which are located close to the nail bed of the finger. Best of all, tapping helps to calm the energy system of the body, even if you're not focused on anything specific.

Tapping on or pinching the nail beds of the fingers helps to 'tone' the energy system of the body. The benefits accrue over time. You can use it to:

- Tap purposefully to release stress and anxiety.
- Tap in a triggering situation to feel more in control.
- Tap away mindlessly to tone the energy system.

CHAPTER 18:
GOT THE SYSTEM?

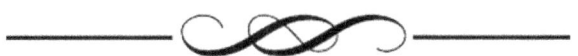

*E**motional healing isn't just first aid. Seemingly minor scrapes in childhood are traumatic to the Child who had to endure them alone. In the Child's mind, he has taken a bullet. When no one is present to soothe the Child and dress the wound, the bullet stays lodged painfully within. Over time it can fester, leading to compulsive behaviors, addiction, and physical dis-ease later in life. Emotional healing is about finding and removing the bullet.* ~ **The Devil's Therapy**

Healing happens the moment the client decides to let it happen. Your job is to create conditions where healing can happen naturally. It happens through a three-phase process of guiding the client into the subconscious mind, finding the emotion coming out of the ISE, encouraging the client to release the feeling, integrating change as it occurs, and testing to see what, if anything, might be left.

The Three Phases

1. Set Up.
2. Transform.
3. Test and integrate.

Phase 1: Set-up.

Phase One is the set-up phase. Ultimately, what you are setting up for is for forgiveness to happen, but the objective of the set-up phase is to prepare the client for the healing process of Regression to Cause therapeutic hypnosis. This is accomplished through the intake process, pre-hypnosis educational process, and during the client's first hypnosis session.

1. Intake process.
2. Pre-hypnosis educational process.
3. Initial hypnosis training session.

Phase 2: Transform.

Phase Two is where the transformational work of Regression to Cause hypnosis takes place. The objective of this phase is to regress to the causal event (ISE), then release everything that has been contributing to generating unwanted symptoms.

The core work of regression hypnotherapy lies in the two Rs in R2CH - regress and release – and the reparenting and re-educating processes of Inner Child Work.

The goal is to find the root of the client's issue and release the problem in the event where it got started. Because every problem is the result of a life experience, regression hypnotherapy focuses on what's generating the client's discomfort – feelings and emotions.

Releasing the thought and emotional energies trapped in the ISE effectively weakens the overall pattern. By clearing the "lesser charge" you'll make the "greater offenses," which occurred later in life, much easier for the client to deal with.

4. Regress to cause(s).
5. Inner Child Work.

Phase 3: Test and integrate.

Phase three is about testing the results and integrating all changes. This is because unresolved aspects can be restimulated by events which, in some way, act as reminders of the ISE. This leaves the client vulnerable to re-triggering.

Once freed from being *stuck* in that specific pattern of perception, the Inner Child will finally be *able* to grow up without the overburden of unresolved thought and emotional energies. This gives you an Adult who can do the forgiveness work required to achieve a lasting change.

The goal is to achieve effortless permanence. This begins by testing the results (a) at the ISE, (b) during the process of growing the Child up through the SSEs, (c) through Future Pacing, (d) in the client's daily life. When this has been successfully accomplished, the client will be ready to do the Forgiveness Work.

6. Test and integrate all changes.
7. Forgiveness Work.

Universal Healing Steps

The 4 Universal Healing Steps[56] give you a simple template you can use at every phase of the healing process. There are a lot of "what ifs" that can arise in a regression session but if you're systematic, and follow

---

[56] The Devil's Therapy: Hypnosis Practitioner's Essential Guide to Effective Regression Hypnotherapy

these steps, you'll always know what the next step needs to be in a session. The client will provide it.

1. Find it!
2. Feel it!
3. Heal it!
4. Seal it!

Find it!

Hypnosis is all about focused attention. What are you looking for? That's where the focus needs to be. For example, if you're facilitating the intake process, what you're looking for is a potential Bridge. Where is the *pain* in the client's story? That's a subconscious signal coming out of the event that caused it.

If you're educating the client about the process, you're looking for conscious and unconscious objections that might block you. What fears or misconceptions does the client have about hypnosis? What about regression? This is an uncovering procedure that you can weave into the intake process. For example, why did they decide to "try" hypnosis? What do they know about hypnotherapy? How do they feel as they talk about past events? Where's the resistance?

If you're guiding a client into hypnosis, you're looking for signs of resistance. Resolve it! You're looking for the "sweet spot" by testing for somnambulism. You're helping the client find the proof they need to know that hypnosis happened.

If you're following a Bridge, you're looking for the first time they ever felt "that feeling". Addressing the problem in the causal event makes the process of facing uncomfortable memories and emotions much easier on the client. This is because the ISE tends to be the event with the least emotional charge. As a result, it's the weakest point in the chain of events responsible for causing the problem.

If you're facilitating Inner Child Work, you're looking for the thoughts and feelings of the Child. That's what is generating the symptoms.

This is where many newbies fail. They think that *uncovering* what happened will resolve the client's issue. Insight is nice, but it won't always change the feelings trapped inside. *That* is what needs to change. We change how it feels by *releasing* the emotional charge.

Here is the secret to getting a lasting change. Release everything – thoughts and feelings – then forgive the Child for holding onto those things. The client needs to recognize that the Child doesn't need to be forgiven because the Child is innocent. The Child is never to blame. With this understanding, the client is ready to experience what it's like to grow up knowing that she's a worthy soul on an important journey and feeling that it's true. As a result, the client can view the opinions of others are simply that – opinions – which have no power because they don't change the Truth about who and what she is.

If you're facilitating Forgiveness Work, you're looking for the thoughts and feelings being harbored by Adult consciousness as grievances toward a specific person. You're looking for an expression of anger. You're looking for a complete releasing of "that anger" to restore internal peace and security.

Feel it!

The way to release a feeling is to feel it. Feel it fully and it will finish and dissolve to nothing. Encouraging the client to release the emotional charge that's been holding the symptom-generating pattern in place will result in greater clarity - physically, mentally, and emotionally. They'll discover that symptoms don't just arise out of nowhere. They have roots in the client's experiences growing up. When an issue is emotional in nature, the cause of the problem lies in an experience that caused that emotion to form in the first place.

What makes any experience memorable is how it feels. Comfortable feelings and emotions are associated with happy memories. Uncomfortable feelings and emotions are associated with stressful experiences in the past. These memories are held onto for future reference and serve the purpose of survival. When left unresolved, painful memories can generate unwanted symptoms later in life. Because the subconscious mind learns through association, the easiest way to facilitate a regression is to keep the focus on feelings and emotions.

Focusing on the specific emotion, that has everything to do with the client's presenting issue, will give you a Bridge right back into the event that caused it. This event set the pattern for responding to similar events in future. Subsequent events which are a match to the ISE then serve to reinforce the underlying pattern, making it stronger.

When the Child comes fully to peace in the ISE, she will be able to move through the traumatic event without being triggered. Nothing has changed except how she feels. As a result, she can observe what happened free of any emotional charge. This is the state we want to *grow the Child up* in. It's a state of Wisdom.

Once you have resolved the energy that's been trapped in the ISE, you can grow the Child up through the SSE's - knowing what she now knows, and feeling what she now feels *as a result* of having had that experience (thus giving it value). Gather up all the changes and instruct the client to take them with her into the next SSE.

As you're growing the Child up, watch closely for triggers in subsequent events and integrate all changes along the client's timeline.

Heal it!

Only what is loving is true. If the client experiences a shift toward feeling better, that's a movement in the direct of self-love. Validate it! Suggestions which are congruent with the client's internal "truth" will automatically be accepted uncritically, reinforcing the newer, better state, and opening the gates to greater clarity.

Think in terms of increments of change. Each newfound level of clarity makes it safer for the client to begin connecting all the dots between "what happened", how that was perceived at that time, what it made them feel, and how that experience culminated in unwanted symptoms. You can't tell them. They must discover it for themselves. Only then is it true.

When the client finally realizes how they've been doing it to themselves in their own mind, that their thoughts have been the cause of unwanted symptoms, they will be empowered to choose differently. When they make newer, better decisions regarding self, others, and life, these choices will be reflected in the client's daily living.

Seal it!

All healing is self-healing. As a result, it can take time. When appropriate, homework can be assigned to support the client between sessions and to test the results. Testing is important because you can't *make* a person heal. All you can do is guide the process.

When the ISE has been resolved, polishing techniques can be used to reinforce, generalize, enhance, and seal in the new pattern. If the client's issue appears to be completely resolved, wrap up their final session with suggestions and imagery to celebrate success, reinforce all the positive changes that have occurred, and build positive mental expectancy for the future.

The Future-Self Test

Prior to emerging, remind the client of the reason they're taking this journey with you by saying, "In a moment, I'm going to count from one to five to bring you back to ordinary consciousness. Before that happens, take a moment to imagine your Future Self is standing right in front of you. Now, step forward into that person and instantly become that person. Notice how that feels. One, you can see the world through the eyes of (e.g., confidence) . . ." Continue emerging count with intermittent suggestions, then on the count of four, "Preparing to open those eyes. But those eyes will not open until you are *convinced* that this is now your reality."

The Gateway Wrap-up

"Imagine that you are standing on a hilltop. Notice that, before you, stands a gateway. Behind you is the path that brought you to this point. Before you lies the path forward. You are standing on the threshold. Before you step through the gateway, pause a moment and review everything it took to get you here. All the learnings. Good times, bad times. All the failures and successes. Times of sorrow. Times of joy.

"The great mythologist, Joseph Campbell, once said that it wasn't until he was well-advanced in life that he was able to look back on the path he had taken and realize that he had been guided by an unseen hand. Look back on your life path and observe it all. Bless it all. Release it all. And when you're ready, step through the gateway. (wait)"

CHAPTER 19: WHAT IF ? ? ?

Q: What if the client seems to be falling asleep during induction?

If you're using a relaxation induction, a client who is sleep-deprived will take advantage of the opportunity to grab some much-needed shut-eye. Some clients are taking medications such as SSRIs which interrupt sleep cycles. As a result, they're not getting the deep sleep they need to feel rested and refreshed during the day.

While the client will benefit from the added rest, they aren't paying you to put them to sleep. They're paying you for a specific result. To achieve that result, you need to get them into hypnosis and then suspend them in that state *before* they drift over into a sleep cycle.

If you suspect that the client is taking a snooze, here's what to do: without changing tonality, say, "In a moment I'm going to count from one to three. On the count of three, let those eyes open. One . . . two . . . THREE."

If the eyes open, they're not asleep. In this case, wave your hand down to give a non-verbal command to close the eyes and give the suggestion to go deeper relaxed. Then, continue with your induction process.

If the eyes do not open, wake the client, and switch to a rapid induction. Remember, hypnosis is the by-passing of the Critical Faculty of the Mind. It doesn't require relaxation. Once you get the client into hypnosis, you can give suggestions for both mental and physical relaxation.

Note: SSRIs disrupt natural sleep cycles. I had a client who was taking two SSRIs who was seriously sleep-deprived. He would drop off to sleep in the middle of an interactive process! In this case, I had him sit upright in the chair to break the association of relaxation to the recliner. I then kept my hand on his shoulder. The moment he started to drift, I would give him a shake and say, "Stay with me! I can't do this without you!"

> *Q: Client is coming for the first time full of anxiety that they won't do it well with hypnosis because they think they can't give up control.*

This is an important part of the setup phase – to remove fears and misconceptions by educating the client about the healing process. I always start the initial conversation by exploring the client's problem and how *they* think hypnosis can help. During this conversation, I want to uncover specific worries or concerns about (a) the hypnosis, and (b) allowing uncomfortable feelings and memories to be a part of the process.

This gives me the information I need to address the client's fears and concerns regarding the process while making the client a partner in the healing process. What the client needs to understand is that the purpose of hypnotherapy is to put them back in charge of some area of their life that they have been out of control to. They don't need to "give up control". They need to *take back* control. Reassure your client! Let him know that you're going to *teach* him how to use this wonderful state to achieve his therapeutic goal. All he needs to do is follow your instructions.

For more detail, read my book: **Ditch the Script**: Get Everything You Need from the Client for Successful Hypnotherapy and Set Up to Wrap Up with Results.

Q: What is your opinion on self-hypnosis, its use, and limitations?

It's been said that all hypnosis is self-hypnosis. This is because the process of guiding a client into hypnosis requires the client's cooperation. It's by following your instructions that they take *themselves* into hypnosis. But many people don't realize that hypnosis is a natural ability we all have. In fact, we go in and out of hypnosis throughout the day. It's called the Basic Rest and Activity (BRAC) cycle. Every ninety minutes or so, our conscious mind takes a little break of about twenty minutes, allowing the mind-body system to "reset". Why not use it?

One of the easiest ways to improve the results you're getting with your clients is to add self-hypnosis as homework to their healing program. Not only is this a way to empower your clients between sessions, but it also gives you a way to track the results.

Once the client has learned how to access the state, you can teach them how to return to the state very quickly and easily, any time they want to. All that's required is the willingness to develop the skill through practice.

Clients who are willing to do their own self-healing work are highly motivated. They're interested in learning how they can create change for themselves and enthusiastic about participating in their own healing. That's your ideal client!

If the client is willing, self-hypnosis makes a great homework assignment. Some clients will benefit from learning a self-healing or coping technique they can use on their own. Most people will benefit from learning how to relax physically and mentally. Simply being more relaxed can help a person to feel more in control of their choices in daily life. Relaxing in hypnosis can help to improve sleep, increase energy during the day, improve mental clarity and memory, enhance immune function and, in general, help a person to feel better physically and emotionally.

Remember, surface issues respond well to surface techniques. Self-hypnosis is a surface technique and can be used to good effect to improve an existing skill (academic, sports), manage symptoms (stress, pain), or reinforce established behaviors (smoking, weight loss strategies.) For stress management, a fifteen-to-twenty-minute practice, once or twice a day, can help soothe jangled nerves and restore mental clarity. Add suggestions to encourage faster results.

Deeper issues are emotional issues which require a deeper technique like Regression to Cause hypnotherapy. Once you have resolved the underlying emotional drivers that cause the client to think, feel, and act in ways they don't like, insights and changes that occurred in a session can form the basis of suggestions which can then be reinforced through self-hypnosis practice between sessions. Once the client's issue is resolved, self-hypnosis becomes a self-empowerment tool they can use for the rest of their life!

Q: When to use direct and indirect suggestions?

Indirect suggestions are used more with Ericksonian style hypnosis while regression hypnotherapy comes straight out of the school of direct suggestion. Indirect suggestions are more of a covert hypnosis technique which can be useful with some clients during the preliminary conversation and induction phases. But once you get the client into hypnosis, you can switch to direct suggestion because the subconscious mind is very literal.

Once you gain access to the subconscious level of mind, direct suggestions are readily accepted. My communication style is direct. I also prefer to test the acceptability of a suggestion before offering it. As a result, indirect suggestions are unnecessary.

Q: What if a client keeps on saying "I don't know" in answer to questions that are asked?

During the setup phase, instruct the client to answer quickly with their first impression or first sense. Then, when they say, "I don't know," you can reply, "I know you don't know. Give me your first sense."

Remember, the conscious mind doesn't know. When it starts trying to figure things out, it will block the process. Answering quickly prevents the conscious mind from stepping in. The first sense or first impression is subconscious communication.

Q: How to deal with transference?

Transference isn't something that is taught in hypnotherapy schools. In psychotherapy, it refers to a phenomenon in which old feelings, attitudes, desires, or fantasies are subconsciously projected onto the therapist. Counter-transference is when the therapist projects onto the client. People routinely project their feelings onto their partners or children. As a result, many relationship issues involve subconsciously displaced feelings. It can also happen in a therapeutic relationship because the therapist takes on a parental role in guiding the healing process.

I don't know if there's any one way to deal with transference. Ideally, you will recognize when it's happening and direct the focus back to the client's issue. With skill, transference can be utilized, but that falls outside of my qualifications.

Bottom line: whatever is going on with the client is not about you. It's about them *unless* you get hooked. If you get hooked emotionally, recognize that your stuff is being triggered and take steps to do your own emotional healing work so that it doesn't have to happen again.

Q: What if the client wants to use the bathroom during a session?

The easiest way to avoid this interruption is to have the client go to the bathroom before you start the session. However, if your client has a weak bladder, this may be unavoidable. In this case, simply have the client open their eyes, still in hypnosis. Remember, somnambulism is a working state for regression hypnotherapy. Somnambulism means walking around while in a state between awake and asleep. That's hypnosis! Send the client off to the toilet and, when they return, do a rapid induction to deepen their state and continue with your session.

Q: What about ideomotor signals?

Ideomotor signaling is a passive process which does not involve the conscious mind. Regression hypnotherapy utilizes the conscious mind in a process that makes the unconscious conscious. The problem is that ideomotor signals offer only "yes" and "no" responses. This is highly restrictive and makes the uncovering procedure excessively time-consuming. And if you're not careful, "yes-no" questions could act as suggestions which lead you down the wrong path. For example, asking, "Does that make you feel angry?" could elicit a "yes" response when the strongest emotion is fear.

Regression hypnotherapy is an interactive process that allows you to target a specific issue. Through this process, the client's verbal responses provide the *specific* information you need to guide the process. For example,

CH: What's happening that you feel that scared feeling in your tummy?

Client: She's giving me "that look." (That look is a trigger.)

CH: What does "that look" make you think? (The scared feeling is anchored to "that look." This question will uncover the cause which is the thought about "that look".)

Where Ideomotor signaling can be useful is as a lie detector. For example, suppose you ask, "Is that true?" And the client says, "No." But the "yes" finger pops up. Clearly there is a conflict going on!

Q: What about Timeline Therapy?

Timeline Therapy is a useful technique that can be employed in a regression session, but it's different from Regression to Cause hypnotherapy.

Timeline Therapy is a dissociative technique and, like any technique, should be used purposefully in a therapy session. Using this technique with every client would be counterproductive because it reinforces the underlying problem of avoidance.

Over ten years of research in memory reconsolidation has shown that the only way to get a lasting result is to review the memory and release the emotion. Find the memory, feel the emotion, heal the trauma, seal in all the changes to effect a permanent change.

Where the Timeline technique might be useful is when a client lands in an event of severe trauma or torture. That's too much! In this case, I would invite them to float up to their timeline so they can view the event from a safe distance. This allows me to keep the client in the event without re-traumatizing them. From a safe distance, I would then conduct the preliminary uncovering work, and release the intensity of energy associated with the shock of that event. Then, once emotional balance has been restored, I would guide the client to associate back into the event. I would instruct them to go to several moments before anything "bad" happens. I would then continue with preparing the Child for "what's going to happen." This is an example of working with the subconscious mind's Prime Directive to keep the client safe.

> **Q:** *When I was doing Timeline Therapy, we always instructed the client to go to the ISE.*

You should know that I'm not a fan of NLP. It took me four trainings to realize it's just not for me! Here's why. First, real regression requires somnambulism. Timeline Therapy does not. Somnambulism gives you deep hypnosis which provides access to deeper emotional content. The more immersed the client is in the emotion, the less chance you're going to have to deal with a confabulated memory.

Second, just because you give the instruction to go to the ISE doesn't mean the client's subconscious mind is going to go there. It will go to the event that feels most pressing or relevant. Old school hypnosis assumes the subconscious mind is the operators "bitch." I dislike that authoritarian approach and choose to make no assumptions. I figure the subconscious knows what the *real* problem is. I want to make it an ally, not "command" it to do my bidding.

Third, Timeline Therapy is a technique. As such, it can be useful. You just have to choose the best tool for the job/client. As mentioned above, Timeline Therapy is a dissociation technique. The *last* thing I want to do is encourage dissociation. That's 90% of the client's problem; either consciously or unconsciously they're trying to *avoid* the underlying cause of the problem.

If you land in a highly traumatic event - e.g., child molestation - the client doesn't have to relive that experience. In this case, you can have them drift up above the event to their Timeline and view the event from a distance. You're not avoiding the memory. You're just providing enough safety for the client to *face* the truth as their subconscious mind has it *without* re-traumatization. The important suggestion to offer from this perspective is that "it's just a memory." It's already happened. It's in the past. They're just remembering something that is over and done.

Once you restore emotional equilibrium, you can have the client step into the moment *before* anything bad happens, feeling *fully prepared* with the understanding that (a) it's in the past but (b) there's a Part of them that needs their help. You can then establish dual consciousness to do the Parts Work.

Q: How to detach from your own biases?

I prefer to qualify my clients. If my biases don't align with the client's, we're not a good fit. However, session content is not always predictable and situations in the client's childhood may turn out to be shocking or even triggering for some therapists. This then becomes a challenge of self-management.

If you are unable to stay present to the needs of the client, you need to end the session and refer them out. Then, do your own work to clear the block so this doesn't have to be a problem in future.

Q: Before reading your book, The Devil's Therapy, I did Bridging back more or less by accident, sometimes with the physical feelings like pressure on the stomach, sometimes with the emotion like anger or fear, even changing it, sometimes during the way back to the ISE. In the chapter about Bridging back, when you stick to the feeling as a guide, do you mean the emotion or the physical feeling?

Both. The place we feel our feelings is in the body. Where a lot of hypnotherapists get sidetracked is trying to resolve anxiety. Anxiety is an antsy feeling that is felt throughout the body. It's not an emotion. You need an emotion to Bridge back on. Because "that feeling" is targeted in the stomach, you know you're dealing with an emotion. This means you have successfully found an effective Bridge.

The next step is to name the emotion. Naming the *emotion* gives you a targeted path to follow. The signal coming out of the event that caused it (ISE) is an emotion being expressed through a physical sensation. "That pressure" in the gut might be anger, or fear, or sadness, or something else. For example, "this scared feeling in my stomach". Or "this sad feeling in my gut."

When you start Bridging back, the subconscious mind will likely take you to an event that has a lot of pressure in it. This is seldom the ISE. Here's where you can get sidetracked. When you land in an SSE, you may find other emotions have been added to the mix. Some of them will be quite strong. As a result, the temptation will be to change horse mid-stream. Don't do it. If you're following fear back, stick with fear. If you're following sadness back, stay with the sad feeling. Remember, "that feeling" you're Bridging back on is the Symptom Imperative. It's a pure, unadulterated signal coming out of the ISE. That's the bullseye.

Because subsequent events (SSEs) act as reminders of the ISE, they trigger the causal pattern trapped in the ISE, making it stronger. This is basic stimulus-response. BUT as more and more "stuff" typically gets added to the pattern, you can find yourself dealing with considerable complexity, particularly if you're dealing with a physiological problem.

Like panic attacks, physical issues develop over time. The ISE is never a panic attack. Nobody gets cancer first. There's always a history of issues leading up to the diagnosis.

In short, the most effective Bridge is a two-fer. Pair (a) targeted sensation in the torso (throat, chest, gut), and (b) a named emotion (fear, anger, sadness, something else) and stay with it until you locate the event that caused "that feeling."

__Q:__ What if the client sees only colors? The client was mostly finding herself floating in "space" surrounded sometimes by purple, blue or white color. Although we were bringing up the emotion/feeling that we were working on, and following it to the "first time", she kept finding herself floating, surrounded by one of these colors and couldn't go in another direction.

"Floating" indicates that your client has either gone to the womb or the pre-conception space. In this case, I would utilize proprioception. Proprioception is an aspect of perception that identifies our position in space. For example, "First sense – does it feel like you're standing, sitting, lying down, or something else?" If the client answers, "lying down," the next question would be, "First sense- what might you be lying on?"

The key is to chunk down, keep the client tuned in to her first sense, and use the client's adjectives to amplify perception. If the client says, "Floating", the next question would be, "Is that feeling that you're floating a comfortable feeling or an uncomfortable feeling?" If it's an uncomfortable feeling, grind down to the emotion. Where does she feel that uncomfortable feeling in the body?

If she's feeling comfortable, ask, "Where might you be that you're floating comfortably?" or "How young might you be that you're floating comfortably?" If the client says that she is, "little", you have most likely regressed to infancy. At this point, it would be safe to say, "Okay, Little, I'm going to ask you a kind of weird question . . . Does it feel like you're *inside* Mom or *outside* Mom?"

Usually, this question will bring the scene into full awareness but, if the client says, "Inside", you'll know she's gone to the womb. If she says, "Outside Mom", the next question would be, "Where is Mom that you're floating?"

Alternatively, you could instruct the client to stretch out her senses and explore the colors. For example, "Where are these colors located?" (Are they inside the body or outside the body?) Is there one color that stands out more than the others? (Isolate one aspect to work with.) How does that color make her feel/think? (Find the feeling.) Is that a good feeling or a bad feeling? Where in the body does she feel "that feeling?" (Zero in on the emotion.) If that feeling could speak, what would it say? (Name the emotion.) Does that color feel new or familiar? (Familiar? Bridge back on it!)

To isolate one color to work with, invite the client to notice if there is a color that seems different or that calls to her. Then have her focus on "that color" and notice what's there or not there. Let the client do the work. If the client has gone to a pre-conception space, it won't be long before she realizes where she's at. In this case, you're all set up to work at a higher dimension.[57]

The most common problem is that clients expect to see. But information isn't always stored visually. For example, infants are still developing their visual acuity. They see things in a diffuse way. But they're very aware of sounds around them, and feelings and sensations in the body. To get more information, you can invite the client to stretch out with her other senses. For example, become aware of the sounds around you – what do you notice?

To tune into physical sensations, ask, "How does that make you feel – comfortable or uncomfortable?" Then, dial down to, "Where in the body do you feel that feeling?"

During a past life regression, I landed in an experience where all I could see was swirling shades of black. That's it. By stretching out with my other senses, I soon realized that the swirling black was water. I soon realized that it was nighttime. I was outside, swimming in black water. From there, the rest of the scene took shape.

---

[57] Gerald Kein called this Ultra-Height.

> *Q: I'm going back through The Devil's Therapy and moving through the Ready for Regression First Session Course, and I just want to clarify something. It appears when you first do regression, you instruct the client to go back to the "first time" they ever felt this feeling. Is that correct?*

The goal of regression hypnotherapy is to locate the "first time" the client ever felt "that feeling." That's the ISE. However, when you're Bridging back, the "first time" is often a Bridge too far. The subconscious mind will tend to go back to an event that has a stronger emotional charge trapped in it because it wants relief. The problem is that this is almost always an SSE. The solution is to use the Lily Pad approach.

Instead of shooting for the "first time", give the instruction to go back to an *earlier* time the client felt "that feeling." When the client lands in an event, conduct the preliminary uncovering procedure to find out what's happening. You don't need a lot of detail. Just get a sense of where they're at, what's happening, who they're with, and what age they might be during that event. Then, test for the ISE using the Feeling Test. (Is that a new or familiar feeling?)

Regardless of what the client tells you, give the instruction to go back to an *earlier* time they felt "that (scared) feeling." Stay with "that feeling" and follow the lily-pads back to the ISE.

The situation where I might give the instruction to "go to the *first* time you ever felt that (scared) feeling" would be if the client has regressed into an event at an early age in childhood. For example, if the client has regressed into an event at age two-years, it's a relatively short hop to locate the ISE. You're virtually sitting on top of it. Note: the veil of forgetting occurs around three and half years of age. If you're *before* that age, the Child will have recall of the ISE.

The *reason* we instruct the client to go to an *earlier* event has to do with the length of the timeline. The older the client is, the further the distance, and the more likely they're going to get lost – *particularly* if you have a weak Bridge. This is where most newbies have trouble – the client loses the feeling. Another reason for regressing to an "earlier event" is to make note of several SSEs so you have a path to follow when it comes time to grow the Child up to adulthood.

It's all about *set up*. You're always setting up for what needs to happen next. **The Devil's Therapy** gives you three phases and seven specific steps to follow. Phase 1 is setting up for Phase 2. Phase 2 is setting up for Phase 3. In Phase 2, we want to follow the Bridge back to the ISE, making note of *subsequent* events that contributed to *growing* the problem, over time. For the record, I have seldom had a client revisit fewer than three SSEs.

In **The Devil's Therapy**, the section on Session Mapping describes how to create a visual representation of the client's timeline. You can then make note of the information associated with each SSE.

Once you locate the ISE, you will have a visual storyline of how the problem got started, how it developed the SSEs and, in some cases, where the problem poked its head above ground in the SPE. When it comes time to grow the Child up just follow your Session Map to reverse the process through which the problem developed to begin with.

Q: Would your ideal client go directly back to the ISE?

The question is – do you always have to find the ISE? The answer is – no. You're dealing with a pattern that was established in an experience earlier in life that is still causing the client distress. That needs to change.

The reason we shoot for the ISE is because it's the event with the smallest emotional charge. There really is only one universal ISE and that has to do with the belief in the separation from God/Source/Universe/Love or whatever word your client uses for their concept of whatever Power created them. All subsequent experiences of insecurity are reflections of this. Fortunately, we don't need to go there because we live in a holographic universe and not everybody is going to embrace the whole God-thing.

There's also this thing I call the Backwash Effect. If you release enough emotional pressure in SSEs, it can backwash into the ISE and neutralize it. Remember, we can ripple positive change forward and backward along the timeline. That means that, theoretically, you could do all the corrective work in the birthing experience. This is another advantage of using the First Session Protocol - if you can get the client back to the womb, you're all set up to do exactly that.

Your approach really depends on the individual needs of the client. I tend to work organically and go wherever the client's subconscious takes us. If we land in the womb, I'm going to spend some time there. If we land in a painful childhood event, I'm going to work from there because *that* is what the client's subconscious mind feels is important. By bringing me to a specific event that has everything to do with "that feeling", it's effectively showing me the "owie."

Q: How do you identify and use a client's "hot" words? By this, I mean, words or phrases which hold significant emotional charge and meaning for the client and can trigger strong emotional responses.

A trigger word or phrase has a personal association to a specific life experience which generates a specific response. Remember, feelings don't come out of nowhere! Something had to happen to cause that feeling. That "something" is the ISE. That's where we work! When it comes to regression hypnotherapy, unless the client is feeling overwhelmed, the stronger the emotional charge, the better!

To identify:
- Watch the body!
- Use Stems Completion Sentences to grind down to the emotion for Affect Bridge. For example, "The thought "snake" makes me feel . . .".

To utilize:
A client's "hot" word can be used to stimulate the emotional response that has everything to do with the presenting issue. For example, I had a client who was so triggered by snakes that she couldn't say or write the word "snake." We had to play twenty questions just to identify what her issue was. Words that sounded like "snake" or in any way reminded of her of snakes – for example, "shake" or "slither" – would cause her to abreact.

It's not the word that's the problem. It's the thought. Words conjure images. That's what a thought is. Standard phobia treatment utilizes this by having the client imagine a situation where "that feeling" associated with the phobic response would be triggered. For example, a client suffering from claustrophobia might imagine stepping into an elevator. This will bring up the emotional response you need to regress into. Remember, we don't want to trigger a panic attack. We just need to find out what the trigger is so we can pull the plug on it!

Regression to Cause therapeutic hypnosis revolves around the two Rs – release and regress. The question is: "Should I regress or release?" The answer to this question depends on where you're at in terms of the three phases in the healing process, as well as the intensity of the client's emotional reaction. For example, in Phase 1, the focus would be on teaching the client how to release the feeling because providing proof to the client that they can feel better instills confidence in the process. In this case, you don't have to resolve everything – just show the client that they're in control of how they feel and that it's possible to feel better.

In Phase 2, on the other hand, the goal is to release the trapped emotions in the event responsible for causing them. In this case, you would need to release everything to get a lasting result.

A strong emotional response is a powerful signal that can give you a Bridge back to the ISE. If the client's strong response occurs during the uncovering procedure, releasing it will reduce internal pressure resulting in greater mental clarity. If the client is overwhelmed by too much emotion, the task becomes to provide safety. To provide safety, you can pause the event, use a dissociative technique, or get the client out of the scene. It all depends on the client.

"Hot words" can also be charged with positive associations. What makes them "hot" is when they're too much. Young children do not have the ability to regulate their emotions. For a developing emotional system, extreme feelings of happiness or excitement can feel overwhelming. This can result in a person putting a lid on their "good" feelings to avoid feeling overwhelmed, again.

You can also reframe negatively associated words to convey a more empowering meaning. For example, I had a client who habitually used the word "whatever" as an expression of disdain. This gave her a sense of control. As we released the underlying feelings of insecurity, I began to incorporate "whatever" into my session wrap up to compound specific changes that had occurred through the healing process. For example, "From now on, *whatever* happens, you're in control." As you can see, the client provides the information you need to guide the process.

> *Q: During the intake conversation, the client identified some of the big SSEs. But I didn't want to take them through any of those SSEs, if we could help it, until we had cleared all the emotion at the ISE which, as you know, is often less traumatic than the SSEs. What's the best way to proceed, in this case?*

The Intake Process is "uploading" the data connected to the underlying problem. When did the problem get started? When did the client first become aware of the symptoms? For example, when did they have that first cigarette?

The first cigarette is not the ISE. It *could* be the SPE, but what a consciously remembered event gives you is a *launch pad* for the regression that has a shorter path to the ISE.

In this case, what you can do is:

1. Induce somnambulism.
2. Do a directed regression to the earliest *consciously remembered* event. e.g., the first cigarette.
3. Conduct the preliminary uncovering procedure in that event to locate the appropriate emotion for Affect Bridge. e.g., what feeling is driving the need to put that cigarette in their mouth?
4. Conduct the Feeling Test for the ISE. (It's not the first time they ever felt "that feeling".)
5. Bridge back to an "earlier time" they felt "that feeling."
6. Follow the Lily Pads back until you locate the ISE.

We're using all the same tools and techniques. We're just adapting them to the specific client. The objective is to shoot for the ISE but if the client lands in a big, fat, hairy-scary SSE, I'm not going to continue Bridging back. That would break rapport because the subconscious mind is showing me where the pain and the pressure is coming from. I want to use that to increase trust by releasing some of the pressure.

You don't have to release it all. Just release enough of it that the client comes to the realization, "I *can* feel better." This is a powerful moment of insight that can clear the path to the ISE! Release some of the pressure. Not all. Just enough that you can test for the ISE. Then, ask permission to go back to an earlier time *with the understanding* that you'll *come back* to this event and take care of it.

In other words, you reduce some of the pressure, then keep your finger on the pause button while you go find the ISE. Why? Because all that pressure in the SSE is the result of the Compounding Effect, over time. If you pull the plug in the ISE, a lot of it is going to drain right out of the SSE. As a result, when you come back to that subsequent event, it will be much easier to resolve because you'll be dealing with the residual stuff rather than the accumulated pain of multiple SSEs.

> *Q: Over the last two weeks I've had three clients regress on the Affect Bridge all the way back to before the womb when they were in the pre-birth realm. Once there, one client reported feeling like she was floating freely without a worry or a concern. The other two were angry at having to come into this life. How would you have suggested I handle these?*

Awesome! Great opportunity! Remember, when the client goes back to the womb and is feeling good, you've landed *before* anything "bad" has happened. You can use this experience to "pre-pave" the way for the life that lies ahead. If the client lands at a point "just before" conception, think of it as landing just before the ISE for this life. Grownup consciousness is in observer mode. Child consciousness is the awareness of the physical self. But before these awareness' develop, there is Soul awareness. Soul consciousness is pre-conception. This consciousness exists *before* conception, during gestation, and post-birth. It's there, always. It's the True Self.

Begin with the standard uncovering procedure. Daytime or nighttime? Inside or outside? Alone or with someone? These initial three questions help the client to associate more fully into the experience. Then, dive into the uncovering process. For example, become aware of where you find yourself. What do you become aware of? As you become aware of "that", what feelings are you feeling?

Get a sense of where the client finds herself. What's it like? Good feelings/bad feelings? It's usually a pretty delicious, floaty space. Light or dark? Pre-conception is always light. Sometimes there are lots of colors. Alone or with someone? This question helps to bring awareness to other presences.

Positive feelings? Amplify. Instruct the client to soak up all the good feelings. Pre-conception is often very womb-like. Pour in the suggestions that "this" is her natural state. Put the emphasis on "love and acceptance."

Negative feelings? This isn't unusual. Sometimes, there's apprehension or anger about entering this life because, from a higher perspective, they know what's going to happen. That's good! Release any feelings of apprehension and encourage a sense of curiosity about what might be learned from this "higher perspective." Remember, nothing bad has happened yet. You're *before* the ISE!

Does it feel like they're alone or with someone? Sometimes they're alone. Sometimes they sense others. If there's a sense of another presence, zero in on it. "Notice . . . As you focus on "that presence", what do you become aware of?"

It might appear as a flickering light, a luminous being, an angel, or even a person they know such as a grandparent who passed over. Whoever is there – qualify them. Instruct the client to go inside and, as they focus on "that presence", to notice how they feel. Comfortable or uncomfortable? If the Presence feels comfortable or good, you can use this Presence in the same way you would employ the Grownup to instruct the Soul/Child. This consciousness knows what purpose experiences in this life might serve, what learning might be gained, to prepare the client/Child/Soul before entering this life. What does this Presence want the client/Child/Soul to know? What does it have to say about the client's presenting issue?

If there's discomfort of *any* sort, that presence doesn't belong there. Have the client say to them, "Be gone." In this case, I would have the "look up and notice what's there." This directs them to look to "higher consciousness". The light will be there. You can always instruct them to find it, feel the presence, know that it is always there when they need it. This suggests safety. Restore a feeling of well-being before proceeding.

The pre-conception space is a beautiful place of higher consciousness. Let the client enjoy the state for a few moments before directing her attention toward the life she is about to enter. Have the client notice the "little one inside Mom". Query the Child's expectations with regards to the relationship she will have with Mom. What about Dad?

Ask if these parents were "chosen" and, if so, by whom? For what purpose? If the client recognizes that they chose these parents for a reason, it sets up for the forgiveness work you will conduct later. In fact, you can begin the forgiveness work by questioning their parents' motives. For example, one of the things I discovered during my own regression to pre-conception was that I was wanted. That came as a surprise! I was also surprised at how young my parents were.

Every parent knows that new parents are *bound* to make mistakes! After all, children don't come with the owner's manuals. But clients seldom apply this wisdom to their own parents because they're stuck in the emotions of their Inner Child. If the client realizes that whatever her parents did to cause her harm was merely due to lack of parenting experience, that it wasn't personal, forgiveness happens. As a result, a tremendous amount of the load of anger the client has been carrying will be drained off. This does not mean we are to make excuses for them but only to recognize that, had they known better, they would have done better. As a result, things would have played out differently. But they didn't. Acceptance is the key to authentic forgiveness. It's giving up the irrational hope for a better past.

What *purpose* might the client's parents have agreed to play a part in fulfilling? How might that agreement factor in? Let the client give you the answers. You'll know what to do.

Once you have filled the client with feelings of goodness and well-being, and have completed the uncovering process, you can begin the Inner Soul Work. This is just like the Inner Child Work except that, instead of Grownup informing the Child, the Presence is informing Grownup and the Child. Interesting, right?

Say to the Presence, "You're the Part of (Client) that knows everything about her, isn't that right? You were there before, and you'll continue to be with her, isn't that true?" Then, have this Soul Awareness focus on the Child Inside Mom (in the womb). Ask, "How far along is that little one?" This will give you the age of the child in the ISE.

I like to ask when Soul Awareness enters the Child. I have been told that, prior to around five months, the Soul energy comes and goes. After this time, it merges with the physical self.

Establish that there is love and acceptance for the Child that (client) will become then ask, "Would you be willing to be there for her from now on?" (Higher self will say yes.)

"Will you be there for her *always*?" (Yes.)

"Even during those times when she is *unaware* of your presence (because we all forget sometimes)?"

Ask, "Are there times you will carry her?"

Continue to ask questions to establish the premise that, whatever happens along that timeline, the client is *going to get through it*, that there is a source of protection, love, and support present, at all times.

Once you have established this loving support - i.e., surrogate spiritual parent - ask Soul Awareness all the questions you might ask Grownup of the Child. For example, "Does anything really, really, bad happen? If so, she needs to know that! Tell her! What does she need to know to get through that?"

Once you have completed the process of informing the Child inside the womb, ask, "Anything else?" When the client reports that it feels complete, you can invite Soul Awareness to "move ahead to the point where you merge with the Little One Inside Mom. 3 – 2- 1 – BE THERE. First impression . . . what's happening?"

Once the merging is complete, I like to turn the womb into a spiritual incubator. Bring all the good feelings into the womb and marinade that little baby in the spiritual energies.

If there are "bad things" happening outside the womb - for example, Mom wants to get an abortion, Dad is drunk and yelling nasty things, etc. - create an insulating field around the Child. We're not changing what happened, but the fact is that Mom didn't get the abortion because the client is still here. And this probably isn't the only time

Dad is going to get drunk and say nasty things. But the Child doesn't need to be affected by these things.

If the client is harboring anger toward a parent, that's where the forgiveness work will lie. Just know that where there is anger, there is always love. The Child needs to love and be loved. It's the accumulated burden of anger over a lifetime that is being carried by the Adult client. This is why the final phase in **The Devil's Therapy** is the Forgiveness Work. It's because forgiveness requires facing the person who did harm. Whoever that person might be, they hurt the client and caused them to get stuck in the fears and insecurities of the Child. Once the Child is grown up to adulthood, you will have a grown-ass woman who can stand up to that person and give him/her whut-for. The Child can't do that because expressing anger means risking losing the love.

Remember, anger is a wall. When a loved-one hurts us, we put up a wall to protect ourselves. It's a natural and necessary self-protective strategy in childhood because the Child is vulnerable. And, often, the people who were supposed to protect the Child didn't. Sometimes, they were the perpetrators. The question is – is that anger justified? If it is based on a misperception, it can be released through understanding. If it's based on physical or emotional harm, a deeper technique will be needed. That's what forgiveness work is all about.

What the Child needs to know, is that Mom and Dad have problems – they are not *her* problems. *She* is not the problem. She's good. She's safe. She's a precious Child of the universe on a journey of *learning*. She can observe and learn without being negatively affected by those things. *That* is the suggestion I want to get in. The seed thought that *no matter what happens growing up*, the client is a worthy soul, is safe and protected, and is not merely going to survive. She's going to thrive. She's going to learn, and grow, in strength and wisdom *because* of those things. I want to instill a sense of *curiosity*. This displaces fear.

Now, there's volumes that could be written on this because every client is going to be different. But if you mentally frame the event in your own mind, all you have to do is stick to the basics.

- Grownup is the conscious, thinking mind of the client.
- Pre-Conception/Past Life Personality is the soul consciousness or super-conscious.
- Child is the subconscious, feeling mind which expresses and experiences through physicality.

Once you have done the equivalent of informed Child work in the womb, you can move the client through the birthing process. Instruct the Child to move to just before they're about to be born into this world/present life. This is such an important moment. They're on the threshold, about to be (re)born!

If there are complications at birth, resolve them. There's always fear coming through the birth canal. Bring in Higher Consciousness as a surrogate Grownup to reassure the Child. Alternately, you can have Grownup begin the reparenting work here, reassuring the Child that she's going to get through, that it doesn't last very long, and that Grownup is here for her, now.

Make sure bonding takes place with Mom - even if it didn't. The Child needs to have this experience growing up in life and modern medicine has robbed too many human souls of this source of self-worth and security.

Once the Child is born, bonded, and feeling safe and secure, you can gather up all the positive energies and send them forward along the timeline. Think of this as pre-paving the future.

If you don't have enough time to process the birthing scene, use timeline generalization. Gather up all the good feelings in the womb and send them forward *through* the birthing experience and through all the ages up to adult age of client "Transforming all the times, and all the ways, you ever wanted or needed (courage, love, support, security, whatever fits with the client's presenting issue) It's all in you now."

> ***Q:*** *I'm conflicted about guiding a client through regression. She is so stressed out that she's close to exploding. She claims that she's been like this for years. She's had a ton of childhood and adult trauma and was referred to me by a psychologist. Today, in the first session, which was straight relaxation with convincers, she said that it was the first time in years that she can remember feeling calm. She even held out her hands to show me that they weren't shaking. She's aware that hypnosis isn't necessarily relaxing, and that the aim is to go for the root cause of the anxiety. But it pains me to give her a taste of relief and then take her right into what I know will be emotionally challenging for her. Her mental and emotional health feel really, really, fragile to me. Do you ever intentionally choose to go in a different direction than regression in cases like these?*

This is a client who will regress very easily. She is already half-way there. All you need to do is grab the energy and guide it. Remember, the "volume" of emotion that she's experiencing has been building up, over time. Remember, the problem is a feeling inside that she doesn't like. She's fleeing from "that feeling". The enemy is within. Don't negotiate with it. Go for the jugular.

While you can manage the symptoms, I'm sure her psychologist has been doing a bang-up job on that front. The question is – what is her therapeutic goal? If she wants to be free of "that feeling", she's going to have to roll up her emotional shirt sleeves, suck-it-up-buttercup, and face the truth of what's going on in her subconscious mind. If you want to get her healed, the way out is through. Trying to "technique" it away is like painting over rusted metal. It won't give you a lasting result.

Trust me when I say this – the client is stronger than you think. The only thing you are dealing with is a memory. It's in the past, and whatever happened, no matter how awful, she's already lived through it. Remind her of this. It's just a dream, a story she's been telling herself, over and over again, in the privacy of her own mind. The problem with talk therapy is that it involves a repetitive regurgitation of undigested emotional material. This reinforces the underlying problem, making it worse.

The reason we shoot for the ISE is because the problem has been building up a head of steam over many, many years. The "first time", however, is the weakest link in a long chain of events. As a result, it has the least energy on the emotional Richter scale. That said, if the client has a bag full of consciously remembered experiences of abuse, you could consider a slightly different approach. It all depends on what happens in the next session.

It sounds like you have established a contract that gives you permission to go where you need to get the healing. You've proved to the client that you can help her find relief. The client emerged from her first session feeling better than she has in years. You have laid the foundation for success. Start the next session with a preliminary check-in and see what comes up. You may find a triggering event that you can use as a launch pad for regression.

Remember, "anxiety is merely a label. If you try to work with "anxiety", you'll spin your wheels. You need to grind down to find the underlying emotion. Anxiety is either fear or anger. Often, it's both. When anger is repressed, it generates depression. This is why anxiety and depression are bed fellows.

Pay close attention to "who" is the source of her pain. Forgiveness Work will be the critical final step to putting an end to the trauma-cycle.

If things went well between sessions, I would probably use the same approach as in the first session and incorporate a positive regression back to the womb. Load the subconscious mind with all the positive thought and emotional energies and send them forward along the timeline.

If you conduct an abreactive regression therapy session that leads into a big hairy, scary event, go *after* the event to drain off the energy. Clear everything in hindsight. Then, once the client is stabilized, go *before* the event to inform the Child before proceeding through the event. You'll find that the emotional intensity will be significantly reduced using this approach.

Another approach is to use a dissociative technique. For example, you can have the client float up above the event and view it from a safe distance. You can place the event in a bubble, a glass jar, or behind a window. If it's still too triggering, fog up the window with steam and invite the client to wipe an area to allow viewing of the event. This provides a sense of control.

Improvise. So long as you have Grownup present, you're good to go. You just have to protect the Child. That's where the emotional energy is trapped. If Grownup is feeling overwhelmed, that will only make things worse. Pause the event and do what you need to do to restore balance. If it's too much for the client, get her out and use talking and tapping to release "what just happened."

> *Q: If I do a positive regression back to the womb, then send her forward along the timeline, am I amping up the original affect to Bridge forward on?*

If the client seems particularly fragile, I would take her back into the womb for the purpose of ego-strengthening. That's what's needed. You need a courageous Grownup, a warrior spirit, willing to step in and guide the little one who was traumatized.

Do the standard uncovering procedure to make sure that the womb is a safe and secure place for the Child. Then, uncover all the goodness. Amplify it. For example, the warmth, the security, the comfort, the safety, and all the good feelings she has for herself. Remember, the Child has no awareness of what's coming. That's Adult awareness. The Child only knows the truth of Now.

The Moment Now that you're looking for is like going before the ISE only, in this case, it's a moment where the *only* thing the Child knows is well-being and self-worth.

If the client is spiritual, find the connection to God/Spirit/Divinity and strengthen it. Employ suggestions to remind the client that this connection is always there no matter what happens. Marinate the Child in this knowing.

You can do a little pre-emptive work if it seems appropriate. Ask the Child in the womb to stretch out with all her senses and become aware of Mom. What does she become aware of? If there's something disturbing there, deal with it. Then, switch to Dad. Stretch out all her senses to Dad. What does she discover? Release an *anticipatory* fear. This will bring down the volume on her anxiety.

Once you have saturated the Child in the goodness, send all the positive thought and emotional energies on ahead along her timeline. You're not growing the Child up, in this case. You're sending a "frequency" out of the womb (like an ISE) to subsequent events. This will change them. It doesn't change what happened in the ISE, but it will install an awareness that was missing the first time. That's pretty much all we do, anyway, right? We release the blocks to allow a more adult awareness to influence the thoughts and feelings of the Child.

I wouldn't rush the womb experience. Time spent there can yield spectacular dividends. If you have lots of time, you can have Grownup step in and inform the Child about what it's going to be like growing up with Mom and Dad (and anyone who has been identified as a perpetrator). Take Grownup off on the sidelines and say, "(Child) can't hear this." Then ask, "Does anything really, really bad happen?"

If Grownup says, "yes", then you need to establish an agreement that the Child needs to know this. Remember, it's the shock that locks in the trauma. Knowing what's going to happen ahead of time diffuses it. Releasing the energy of any anticipatory fear resolves the shock factor. (Review the SEAL Pattern. This is what you need to know to prepare the Child for "what's going to happen.")

The worst part is that Child had to face the experience alone. You can change that. Let her know that this time, Grownup is going to be there with her. Then, have Grownup inform the Child, and reassure her, that she's going to get through that experience.

In situations of abuse, the Child often thinks, "I'm going to die." You can erase this interpretation by having Grownup tell her, "You get to grow up." You can then reinforce this by giving the suggestion that grownup is *proof* that she gets to grow up!

Test to make sure that the Child believes Grownup. If she doesn't, here's a little trick you can use. Have Grownup take the Child with her and show her what life is like as a Grownup. Show the Child all the *good things* she has to look forward to. Hope heals.

If you have gobs of time, progress to the "first time" she ever knew what it was like to feel (specific emotion) or bad in any way. Then test to make sure it's the ISE. She may bounce ahead to an event that has more energy in it. That's okay. Just conduct the test and regress back to the ISE. Then, you can pull the plug on the core emotions feeding into subsequent events.

> *Q: I wanted to ask you something that I never had a chance to ask Jerry when he was still alive and that still puzzles me: when you regress your client, and you are almost 100 % sure that you hit the I.S.E., most clients at that point are clueless about how major what you both discovered is. Do you need to point this out to them? For example, "See, dear client this is major, we just found out the cause of most of your problems!" Some other approaches to hypnoanalysis claim that just by releasing it, the problem is solved, but we Omni people want to maximize the results and now I think that it is better to make sure the client understands the importance of what they just discovered. How would you address that?*

Clearly, some clients are not as insightful as others. This is the challenge of the hypnoanalysis process. Insight is not always necessary – but it sure helps to achieve a complete resolution of the problem. Regression to Cause brings to light the causal event. Hypnoanalysis is the process of bringing to awareness how that event seeded the presenting issue. Hypnotherapy is the process of clearing the underlying cause of the presenting issue.

Many hypnotherapists believe that simply bringing the ISE to conscious awareness is sufficient to resolve the problem. Sometimes, that's all that's needed, perhaps because the client manages to "connect the dots" to the presenting issue and, as a result, is willing to let go of the problem. Clearly, this is not always the case.

Many hypnotherapists think that telling the client that the ISE is the cause of their problems will resolve the problem. But that's just not true. Hypnoanalysis is a process that we facilitate to generate insight into how the ISE caused the event. As the answers lie within the mind of the client, you cannot do this for them. The client needs to discover this for themselves for it to be true.

If you say to the client, "See? We just found the cause of most of your problems!" you're offering a suggestion. If the client does not see it for himself, that suggestion will be rejected. In the absence of belief, there will be no change. This is because there will be no *reason* to change.

Now, I understand that this may seem rather odd when you consider that the conscious mind is the logical, rational, thinking part of the mind. You might wonder, "But if we set aside the conscious mind during the regression, what purpose does reason and logic serve during a regression?" The answer is simple. The Child in the ISE is the conscious mind of the client *at that age*. You are always dealing with the conscious mind.[58]

Because children lack emotional maturity, the ISE embodies conscious decisions which may have no basis in truth or fact. This is what the client needs to recognize. Reality-check the perceptions of the Child by asking Grownup, "Is that true?"

Is what the Child is thinking true? If it is true, then what needs to happen for the Child to get through the situation without being negatively impacted?

---

[58] These are the rings of the tree I describe in **The Devil's Therapy**.

Do you see how this hands responsibility over to the client to find their own solutions? Through the uncovering and insight process, the client will realize some important facts such as, "I didn't know then what I know now . . . if I *had*, I wouldn't have made those decisions that I've been paying for, ever since," *and* "I don't have to hold onto that thought-feeling-belief any longer because *I'm not a child anymore*. I'm a grown-ass adult and I can make better decisions for myself!"

That's a moment of empowerment. When the client gets this, they can educate their Inner Child and, as a result, embody those changes. This is when miracles happen.

Q: What if the client is super harsh with their inner child, starts yelling at them for being incompetent and stupid, etc.?

If the client regresses into an event in childhood and becomes hostile toward her Inner Child, realize that her Inner Parent is contaminating the scene. The Child doesn't need to hear that garbage! It will only add to the burden of unresolved emotions which are keeping the Child trapped in that event.

I learned this the hard way. Never regress a client to a painful event in childhood until you have verified that they can be a loving support to their Inner Child. The easiest way to avoid this is in Phase 1 while you're setting up for the healing process.

First, watch closely for clues during the intake process. You can learn a great deal by asking, "What was childhood like?"

Explore the client's relationship with her primary caregivers. Parents are internalized as Parts. How might these internalized representations be the underlying cause of the client's presenting issue? For example, a client raised by two critical parents may need to be taught how to be present to the needs of their inner Child.

Does the client have children of her own? Exploring this during the intake will allow you to take a pulse on the client's parenting style.

If the client has never raised children, she may not have developed adequate parenting skills. In this case, you may need to educate her about what every child needs.

What does a Child need?[59]

1. Loving touch such as cuddling, stroking, and comforting.
2. Words of endearment, encouragement, and appreciation.
3. Quality time with undivided attention.
4. Rewards, treats, pleasant surprises.
5. Being able to help others, being helped by others.

My approach is to facilitate a positive regression in the first session. This allows me to gauge the client's attitude toward their Inner Child before we start wading into alligator infested waters. That way, if the client expresses hostility toward the inner Child, the task becomes one of "finding the love". Remember, the answers lie within the client – they're just buried.

If the Adult starts projecting blame onto the Child, something is being added to the event that wasn't there the first time. Your primary job is to work with the subconscious mind by protecting the Child.

---

[59] The Five Love Languages of Children by Gary Chapman

Whatever Grownup is putting on the Child is simply not true. Adding hostility to an already-traumatic experience is only going to make things worse. In this case, I would instruct the client to go back to an earlier time, to an event where *all the Child knows is what it is like to be loved and accepted.* You may have to go back into the womb. In some cases, even further. This is where it's helpful to know what the client's spiritual beliefs are, ahead of time.

If the womb situation wasn't safe or loving, you need a place to go to *find* and download the love. Keep Bridging back until you find an event where the Child is loveable. It's there. Children who are deprived of love don't survive, so there must have been someone or something present to meet the emotional needs of the client in childhood. Who was it? Ask the client, "Was there ever someone in your life who really loved you, for example an auntie or a grandparent?" If there was, the client has a role model for loving, supportive behavior that you can use.

Once this person has been brought to awareness, take the client to a situation in the past where she is enjoying the warm feelings of safety and security associated with that person. Let her hear the words, feel the sensations, and experience the emotions of being unconditionally loved and accepted. In other words, download the positive associations. Then, you can either (a) invite that positive role model to act as a trusted guide/teacher to educate the adult client about what the Child needs, or (b) use the positive role model to reparent the Child.

This is rare but, if there really was no one loving in childhood, find out if there was some*thing* the Child loved. For example, did the client ever have a special pet that she loved? If so, you have a source of warm feelings which can be transferred to the inner Child. I had a client whose only source of comfort as a child was a stuffed toy. I used her beloved toy to restore the client's internal sense of safety and security. This allowed her to re-experience feeling loved which provided a transferable resource when it came time for her to step in and support her inner Child. The key is to craft your approach to the specific needs of the client. Then, let the client do the work!

Q: When I was in training, an instructor was demonstrating a regression with a student. The student volunteered and was very open to experiencing regression. But each time she went into hypnosis (regression, Parts, etc.) she ended up with the angels. She was molested by her father when she was young, and her mother walked in on it; lots of trauma to work with. She was a very open person and was aware of the abuse, and yet, in hypnosis she would go immediately to the spiritual realm. What if the client goes right to the angelic/spiritual realm every time?

This is a classic avoidance strategy. The subconscious mind is doing its job by protecting her from those painful past events. See the chapter on spiritual issues for strategies you can apply when this happens because, sooner or later, it will!

Q: I had a client who regressed into a scene where her father was humiliating her in front of her mother and sister by making her stand up and repeat, "I am stupid", over and over, again. Her mother and sister did nothing. The client came right out of hypnosis, sat up and said she never wanted

> *to think about that ever again and left. I kept telling her, via phone, and text, that I could help her neutralize that scene, but she never would come back. What could I have done?*

When a client tries to duck out of an uncomfortable memory, that's resistance. Realize you're right where you need to be. The client's own mind has taken her into a situation that has everything to do with her presenting issue and *consciously* the client doesn't like it. As a result, your client tried to hijack the session by emerging herself from hypnosis. But consider this: at the end of a session, following the emerging count, when the client opens her eyes, she's still in hypnosis. You have a 90-second interval where the client's mind is still wide open to accepting suggestions.

If the client opens her eyes while immersed in a painful emotion, realize she's in **deep** hypnosis! Don't allow her to emerge. Take her deeper into the feeling. "Stay focused on that feeling!"

Keep the attention on the uncomfortable emotion and exacerbate the discomfort. For example, when the client's eyes open, work quickly! Use a slightly authoritarian tone, point to your eyes, and say, "Look right here!" (Focus attention.) Then say, "Well, now we know. Your subconscious mind has just shown us where your healing lies! Thank you, Subconscious! Realize . . . *that situation* has everything to do with (presenting issue) and all the symptoms. This is your miracle moment!"

When a client doesn't want to face a specific event, this should tell you that you're on the bullseye. The problem is that there's a significant emotional charge trapped in that event. The client knows this! But avoiding it isn't going to get her healed because that event has everything to do with her presenting issue! Bottom line: if you let the client take charge of your session, you're sunk. You can try to dance around her issue – in which case, nothing will change – or you reinforce the contract that says, "We go where we need to go to *get the healing.*"

To accomplish this, I would first validate the client's feelings of apprehension. Of course she doesn't want to face that! Who would? What happened in that situation was awful! Nobody should ever have to go through what she went through! But the fact is - it happened. We can't change that. But we can change how it feels and that changes everything.

The client needs to understand that there's an important Part of her that's been stuck in that event. It's *still stuck* in that situation and needs help. This is why her subconscious mind has shown us this event – it knows that you can help! I would work on establishing permission to take her back to *before* anything "bad" happens in that event.

Remember, you need a contract that allows you to do your job. What the client needs to recognize is that avoiding the past is what has been keeping her stuck in the pain of the problem. The subconscious mind holds all our memories. While the conscious mind can forget, the subconscious mind never forgets. As a result, when an experience is left "hanging" like this, situations in daily life can act as reminders of that unresolved painful experience. (The client knows this is true.)

When that happens, either consciously or unconsciously, the person gets triggered. This causes the whole emotional pain package to be re-experienced. That's what a panic attack is. Every time we're triggered, not only do the feelings trapped inside bubble up to the surface, but they also grow stronger. This is due to the compounding effect. As a result, problems tend to get worse over time.

Like it or not, she's reliving that event over and over, again. You can put an end to the reruns. To "mop up" after the fact, one option might be to use a modified Fork in the Road metaphor to review where the client has been and now finds herself. She's facing a choice.

On the one hand, there's the past and all the consequences of holding onto those painful feelings, i.e., symptoms. That's the bad news.

On the other hand, "Now you know . . . that situation has everything to do with the (presenting issue)."

Provide the conscious mind with a reason for "that feeling" by reminding the client of how that situation has impacted her for her entire life. "That feeling" is the reason she's seeing you! Something happened to motivate her to come to you for help, right? Remind her of that. For example, "Think of everything you've tried to get rid of this problem. You've *tried* running from it. Lord knows, you've *tried* to forget about it. But it's still there, in the back of your mind, day in and day out, controlling you (and you know that's true) . . . controlling how you feel about yourself, and robbing you of your good feelings about yourself. You've carried this long enough! This is the moment where everything changes . . . or nothing changes. It's up to you."

To resolve the problem requires the client's permission because you can't do it for her. After all, it's *her mind*! Employ a little 'rah-team' coaching. And let her have the power to decide how to proceed. For example, "There's a brighter future waiting for you, on the other side of this. That's why you're here! On some level *you know* that the way out is through. The good news is that you don't have to face it alone, like you did the first time. We do this together. Realize you're not a child anymore. You're a grown-assed woman! The problem is that your subconscious mind doesn't know this, yet. There's nothing back there that you haven't already lived through. If you can face it and feel it, you can heal it. Then it's over."

The client needs to be willing dig in, and dig down deep, to find the courage needed to face what's there. Remember, all you're dealing with is a memory! That experience is in the past, but her subconscious mind doesn't know this! Remind her, "Back then, you were just a kid. You didn't know how to deal with it. As a grownup, you have more experience to draw from. The problem is that your subconscious mind thinks you're still a child. We need to change that – so you can heal!"

Remember, every problem is the result of a life experience. She needs to be willing to face that 800-pound emotional gorilla that's been controlling her life and take back her power. This is where the work lies - in resolving the client's resistance to facing and feeling the underlying cause of her unwanted symptoms. Provide safety by reminding her, "You had to face that situation, all alone. *This time*, it's going to be different! *This time we will do it together.* And we take no prisoners! Deal? (Establish willingness.) It is time to take back your power and set yourself free of the past! *Ready?*" (Establish the contract.)

If the client is not willing to follow your instructions, there's nothing you can do. In this case, I would leave the contract open. Remind her that while *it's possible* to be free of the past (you know this because "we do this all the time") you can't do it for her. When *she's ready* to face her truest feelings, you'll take care of it. When that event is finally put where it belongs - as a worn-out, faded memory - it will have no further power to control how she thinks or how she feels, and her whole life will change for the better. Then ask, "What's it going to be? You decide."

If the client is still resistant to regressing back into the event, I would focus on clearing what the client remembers consciously. Titrate the event and use past tense to clear all the consciously remembered aspects. This will drain off a tremendous amount of internal pressure and, with it, much of the client's resistance. As a result, you may gain permission to take the client back to before the event to prepare the Child. In addition, you'll have a much more resourceful Grownup to work with. Win-win.

To facilitate the clearing process, I would start with a general statement such as, "Even though I was shamed and humiliated as a kid/ and *I can still feel it/* I don't have to feel this way for the rest of my life/ because I deeply and completely accept myself." (Reminder phrase, "This *shameful humiliation* . . . in my (gut/heart/throat)."

Notice how you can use an event title to depersonalize shame? Instead of taking on shame because of what he did, you can reframe it as shameful behavior. Humiliating an innocent child is a "shameful" behavior. That is wrong. The Child did nothing to deserve that treatment. There's nothing wrong with the Child. The Child is innocent. Do you see how these suggestions open the door to self-forgiveness? All forgiveness is self-forgiveness.

To process the consciously remembered event in hindsight, invite the client to tell the story from the beginning using past tense. Titrating the event allows you to chunk down and deal with one perception, one thought, and one feeling at a time. The moment the client bumps into an uncomfortable feeling *everything stops*. Pause the scene and release that feeling. This will ensure that the client doesn't get overwhelmed.

When you get to the end of the story, celebrate "getting through it", then rewind to the beginning (knowing what you now know), and tell the story, again. Wash, rinse, repeat until the entire event has been neutralized.

You can then invite the client to go back *before* the event. With her permission, guide her back to "before anything bad happens" and review the event to test for any residual aspects. If there is still an emotional charge around that event, regress back to an earlier time. Resolving the "first time" she ever felt that feeling would effectively pull the drain on all subsequent events, thus reducing the pressure.

Remember, shame and humiliation are thoughts. Make sure you're dealing with an actual emotion. i.e., fear, anger, sadness which is targeted in the torso region (throat, chest, gut.) Shame is a thought that says, "I'm bad to the bone. I have no intrinsic value. Might as well go eat worms." Humiliation is a response to a perceived attack.

The source of attack, in this case Dad, is best dealt with in the final step of Adult Forgiveness because the Child is still feeling vulnerable and scared. However, if it seems appropriate, an alternative approach would be to provide a safe place where the can be herself. E.g., Gray Room.

Establish a suitable seating arrangement for the dialogue process, then bring Dad in. I would duct tape him to the chair and gag him so that he can't do or say anything. This puts the client in control and may even give her a perverse sense of pleasure.

Once you're set up, invite the client to say everything she couldn't say to Dad as a Child. For example, tell him how that experience affected her. What did he make her think? How did he make her feel? Tell him how it's *still* affecting her. Purge the emotions. Give him back all his false beliefs and negative emotions. Reclaim everything he took from her as a Child. Then, go for forgiveness.

When forgiveness is complete, you can have the client review the scene to test the results. Then, see if the client can find some learning in having had that experience that can empower her, from now on. Grow the Child up through the SSEs in that knowledge and wisdom. Integrate all changes at the adult level of consciousness. Future pace to test and reinforce the client's vision for a newer, better future.

> *Q: What if a demon shows up and takes them over and begins speaking? This actually happened during one of my sessions!*

Been there. Several times. Spirit Releasement Therapy is a specific therapy that can be integrated into regression hypnotherapy, but there is too much to it to cover here. What you'll find is that these "hitchhikers" are always congruent with the client's beliefs. For example, if the client was raised in a family system spewing punishment, fire and brimstone, demons are real!

Recognize you're dealing with a spiritual (belief) issue. Most of the time you're not dealing with an actual demon. (If you are, you'll know it! In this case, you need to be prepared.)

Most of the time, you're dealing with a Part of the client that has been rejected, amputated, abandoned, and/or abolished. What this should tell you is that the client is carrying a considerable load of fear and self-hatred. My approach to dealing with these "nasty players" is to accept that they are what they say they are until I can find a way to prove otherwise. To accomplish this, I play dumb and ask lots of questions. (It frustrates the hell out of them!) For example, ask, "How long have you been with (client)? How old was she when you joined her?" This question gives you a target for regression.

You can ask the Part to "show you" by taking you back to the event where they "joined" with the client. Remember, Child Parts are feeling Parts. Keep following "that feeling" back until you find the ISE.

Ask, "Who hired you?" (If they don't know, it's not a demon. If they don't want to tell you, recognize that they're scared. Probe gently.)

Ask, "What's your purpose?" Then, "What happens if you don't fulfill your purpose?" The purpose of this question is to uncover guilt. (Demons - even the confabulated ones - always work for the devil. Their job is to punish the client by making life a living hell.) Guilt is anger directed toward oneself. That's a self-punishment program.

Ask, "What does she need to be punished for?" This can help to identify the event that is calling for forgiveness. (It can be helpful to express pity and point out that they're stuck in a dead-end job that offers no benefits.)

Ask, "What happens if you don't do your job?" If they don't know, that's fine. Recognize that the Part is confused. Perhaps the Part served a useful purpose at one time, but now it has lost the plot. This may open the door to negotiating a new job or purpose that is better suited to the needs of the Part and the client. (In other words, standard Parts Therapy approach.)

If the Part tells you that failure to do their job will result in being sent to the pit, find out what they know about the pit. What's it like? Have they ever been there? How do they feel about "that place." Usually, it terrifies them. There's the fear! Poke around a little to grind down to the specific fear. Performance fear? Fear of punishment? Fear of failure? This will give you a targeted signal to follow back to the ISE.

Often, these Parts are afraid of the Light. They have been told that the Light will destroy them. Ask, "Who told you this?" Reality check this. "Is it true? How do you know it's true?"

Recognize this as a Part of the client that has been cut off from the love and forgiveness of God. Imagine how awful that must be! Express pity. Find out if they feel sorry for themselves. If so, the door is open for healing. In this case, ask, "If you could change things for yourself, would you?" Don't be surprised if you're told, "It's not possible!" That's where the client is stuck – in the feelings of hopelessness and powerlessness of a child.

A Complex Issue

> *I have a client who has been repeatedly betrayed by close family members resulting in distrust of people who use certain phrases. How do you de-stigmatize these phrases? For example, when someone said, "trust me", it was a lie. If they said, "You can trust me to keep your confidence, they couldn't wait to broadcast it to the world." A sister said, "Believe me", right before draining the client's retirement fund. A sister-in-law said, "Have I ever lied to you?", right before stealing the client's car keys and totaling her car. This*

> *client has been raped, not once, not twice, but three times by different people, and each time was told, "You will absolutely be safe." She heard "I love you for you", right before a wedding proposal which turned out to be an attempt to obtain a green card. "Nothing bad will happen", right before the person tried to smother her with a pillow. "I will pay you back", after fraudulent credit card charges were discovered. She was then stuck with the payments. "I would never XYZ"; meanwhile paperwork was being drawn up to do exactly XYZ and more.*

This is a complex issue because there's an ongoing pattern of betrayal. The problem with betrayal is that it can result in a sort of hypervigilance that becomes a block to intimacy. How can a person ever truly open to another person when past experiences have taught them to expect a betrayal? They're always waiting for the "whammy" which surely must come because, as Gerald Kein said, "What the mind expects tends to be realized." Worse, when the hits just keep on coming, subsequent experiences only compound the underlying beliefs.

A Stigma

Here's what you're dealing with. A "stigma" is an association of *disgrace or public disapproval* with something, such as an action or condition. For example, a person can be stigmatized for being different or for having a limp or a stutter. We call this bullying.

A "stigma" is also defined as a *set of negative and unfair beliefs* that a society or group of people have about something. A belief is a well-practiced thought. The problem is that "bad" experiences establish false beliefs which become self-fulfilling prophecies.

A synonym for "stigma" is *stain*. That's shame. Shame isn't about what was done – it's about who you are as a person. Events of shaming early in life form a part of a person's identity. Betrayal, on the other hand, is an abandonment issue. What do you suppose happens when the people who were supposed to love and take care of the child don't do their job? The child takes the blame.

Untangling the Pattern

What your client is dealing with is an emotional Gordian Knot. While it will require patience and persistence to set her free of the past, what your client needs to know is that her subconscious mind is doing exactly what it was designed to do. Remember, human beings learn from experience. The subconscious mind naturally generalizes all learning so it will know how to keep us safe in the future.

While the subconscious mind generalizes all learning, it is very specific. To untangle this pattern, you first need to identify all the trigger words and phrases.

For example,

- Trust me.
- Believe me.
- Have I ever lied to you?
- You're absolutely safe.
- I love you for you.
- Nothing bad will happen.
- I will pay you back.
- I would never . . .

Find the Feeling

You can then use Stems Completion Exercise to identify the feelings and emotions attached to these words/phrases. For example, "The thought 'trust me' makes me feel (scared, sad, angry) in my (throat, heart, gut)." What emotion is attached to those words? Where in the body does the client feel that feeling?

When a person betrays you, you learn that *they* can't be trusted. *They're* not safe people. You cannot believe what they're telling when they're liars. And when someone breaches confidentiality, you feel exposed and vulnerable. That's fear. When someone flat-out lies to us, we feel angry. That's normal. But when the people who were meant to protect and support you in childhood can't be trusted, how can you trust *anyone*? Worse, how can you trust *yourself*?

What's safe?
Subconsciously "safe" isn't what most people think. Safe is simply "what's familiar." If that happens to be sh*t and abuse – guess what? You're going to gravitate to it. It's not that we "create our own reality." It's that we are attracted to familiar patterns because *that* is what we know how to cope with. This is the fundamental problem that your client is dealing with. She is attracted to people who will betray her because, subconsciously, they are a perfect match for "what's normal."

What's normal? People who aren't trustworthy. Liars. They'll *seem* trustworthy, loving, generous, and honest – at least to begin with - but sooner or later, they turn out to be just like the "last guy." This is essentially what Battered Wife Syndrome is about. It's not that the woman wants a man who will treat her badly. It's that her subconscious mind is trying to come to peace with a corrupted love relationship – usually with a primary parent.

Find the ISE
This is where the answers lie – in childhood – and with the people who *should* have been kind and loving and trustworthy. The events you have

listed here appear to be consciously remembered events which happened later in life. In other words, these are SSEs which could be identified during the intake process and show you the underlying pattern of betrayal which must have happened early in life.

The internal conflict that her subconscious mind is trying to resolve has to do with the fact that this was "normal" in her family of origin. That is where she learned what to expect and what she *deserves* from others and from life. To resolve this, you need to locate the ISE(s) and uncover the specific thought(s) that formed the belief(s) that are keeping her stuck on the merry-go-round of repeating the same-old-same-old pattern.

Clear the Events
Keep in mind that you're dealing with a lifelong pattern of recurring betrayals, not a single event. There will likely be multiple ISEs calling for resolution. However, one ISE can contain several trigger words or phrases. You just need to thoroughly clear each event before moving onto the next one. Clear everything, then test to make sure that there's nothing left before focusing on the next aspect to Bridge back on. As you release the internal pressure trapped in these earliest events, the subconscious mind will start to catch on and generalize these changes to other events. As a result, the client will start to notice changes in the people around her.

Get a Lasting Result
Where you're going to find the lasting result (and end the repetitive pattern) is through the Forgiveness Work. While you're doing the uncovering work, keep a list of all the people in childhood who hurt her, lied to her, betrayed her, treated her like dirt. Then, when you get

to the final step in the healing process, deal with these people, one by one.

If the Adult is holding onto a lot of anger toward these people, start with the person who has the least emotional charge around them. Warm up to the bigger wins. Remember, the subconscious is not the enemy. It has been doing an exemplary job of protecting the client. It's not going to give that up until you prove to it that the client can handle it.

Remember, it's the Inner Child who is still trapped in those events, trying to cope with the crazies in her family, and trying to find a way out of the chaos. This leaves the subconscious mind struggling to resolve this problem because it *only has the resources of the Child in that event*. That's where the work begins.

Once you have a list of every consciously remembered experience of betrayal, pick the situation that occurred at the *earliest age* as a launch pad for regression.

Induce hypnosis and direct the client back to this earliest event. Review the event to find the feeling. Bring up the feeling powerfully for Affect Bridge. There will likely be anger and fear. Follow the fear. Fear is the root of all negative emotions. It's the Child's first response.

Lily pad back until you locate the ISE for "that feeling." Conduct the preliminary uncovering work, then release everything in the ISE that is connected to "that feeling" including things said, things done, and the client's thoughts and decisions about those things.

Remember, the key to effective releasing is clear everything. Don't try to change horse mid-stream. Keep the focus on that one thought/feeling until its zeroed-out. For example, if the trigger phrase is, "Trust me", that's a thought. Release on, "The thought *trust me* makes me feel (scared.)" Note: Distrust is not an emotion. Distrust says that it's not safe to trust. That's fear.

Forgiveness is the Healing

Have Grownup forgive the Child in the event. Even though the Child has done nothing wrong, the client still needs to forgive her. Remember, all forgiveness is self-forgiveness. She's forgiving a Part of herself. Forgive the Child for holding onto the pain for too long. Forgive her for not knowing how to deal with a crazy person. Validate her innocence.

When the Child can move through the event without being triggered, grow her up to adulthood and integrate all the changes at the grownup level of consciousness. Compound all these changes. Remember, as the Child changes, Grownup changes. If the Child feels better, Adult client is going to feel better.

Wash, rinse, repeat.

If there are other events with different people (Offenders), repeat the process. Releasing the energy trapped in the events associated with these people will result in the client feeling tremendously better.

If there are multiple events with the same person, you can sometimes suggest that the subconscious mind merges all these experiences into a single event. You can then clear that theme-based event *as if* it was the ISE.

Adult Forgiveness

When all events have been cleared, the only thing left is to release the grievance(s) the Adult has been carrying around. Draining off the energies trapped in past events will reduce the "volume" of anger you have to deal with. This will make the Forgiveness Work much easier for both you and the client.

Remember, you need a grownup for this part of the healing work. It's grownup that is carrying a burden of unresolved grievances. The Inner Child only has a single event (ISE). There can be multiple events and, therefore, multiple Inner Children, i.e., one for each age/event.

To setup for Chair Therapy with the Offender(s), create a safe place for the client to face "that person". Grey Room, Round Room, Red Room, or the kitchen table are all good options. Establish two chairs facing each other. The client sits in one chair and the Offender sits in the other.

Deal with one person at a time. Start with the least harmful person. For example, a sibling who was close to the same age as the client will be much easier to forgive than a raging father. Forgiving this person will teach the subconscious mind that it's safe to let go of the problem.

Safety is Job #1. If the harm done to the client was especially heinous, duct tape the Offender to the chair. If Offender is mouthy, put a gag on him. Ensure that he doesn't have any power. Let the client know that "that person" can't do anything - all they can do is listen. This gives the client the upper hand in the relationship. Proceed with the Forgiveness process. Release all the anger. Then conduct the forgiveness test.

Remember, Grownup is holding onto the *accumulated* anger. That anger is generating tremendous internal pressure which drives an internal *need* for relief. The way to get that relief is to *purge* the anger trapped inside and then forgive each of the Players, one at a time.

This requires a balls-to-bone level of truth-telling. Client needs to tell "that person" everything that needs to be said, how that person hurt Client when she was just a little girl, why what they did was wrong, and how their behavior has impacted Client for her entire life. The Offender is a dumb ass who needs to be educated. Then, Client can take back her power. The way to do this is through Pillow Therapy. Encourage Client to keep talking and pumping the anger out into the pillow until there's nothing left.

What did you learn? What's one strategy that you can use right away in your healing practice?

FINAL THOUGHTS

In 2003, I had the privilege of being one of five hypnosis practitioners to be accepted into a live training in Florida with the late Stephen Parkhill[60]. I had volunteered to be his 'demo unit' for the class because I was the tenderfoot of the group, with only a few years of practice under my belt, and I had also never experienced an actual regression session, let alone with a world-class healer.

Be careful what you ask for. A few days before I got on the plane to fly to Florida to attend the training, I detected a lump on my breast. The lump was clearly visible and about half the size of my pinky fingernail. As I was unable to get an appointment to see my doctor before my trip to the States, I scheduled the appointment and got on the plane.

On the third day into the course, Parkhill invited me to come up to the front of the class so that he could conduct the demonstration of his approach to Regression to Cause hypnotherapy.

To begin the session, Steve asked me to briefly describe the issue I wanted to work on, and I told him that I had a lump on my breast. After conducting a brief intake, Steve rolled his chair back, leaned

---

[60] Stephen C. Parkhill is the author of Answer Cancer: The Healing of a Nation (Miraculous Healings Explained).

forward, and looked me straight in the eye. "How much of what you just told me is true?" he asked.

"All of it," I replied, "except I haven't seen a doctor."

Parkhill raised his eyes skywards and said, "You never know what they're going to send you! Okay, looks like we're going live, folks!"

With that, he proceeded to guide me through what I can only describe as a breath-taking roller-coaster ride into my past.

The next day the lump was visibly half its previous size.

A week later it was gone completely.

Two weeks later, the lab tests were back from the lab and my doctor delivered the diagnosis – nothing. There was no sign of any problem whatsoever.

I learned a tremendous amount from that session. It showed me, in no uncertain terms, how the subconscious mind can make mountains out of molehills. I have no doubt that what the mind builds can be unbuilt. I am equally certain of this: if you're drawn to this work, it's because you have been called to healing, but it's up to you to prepare yourself for the task by doing your own work.

Honestly, it will make you a better healer. Tools and techniques are great but don't discount the value of first-hand experience. There is much to be gained from putting yourself in the "hot seat" and experiencing the healing process from the inside. My own experience solidified my faith from "belief" to "knowing." This allows me to speak with conviction about the healing power of the mind.

I absolutely *know* that healing happens – when we let it.

I absolutely *know* that all healing is self-healing. No one can *make* you heal.

I absolutely *know* that mind is the builder (Edgar Cayce wrote that.) And whatever the mind makes can be undone.

I absolutely *know* that revivification is about *feeling*, not seeing.

I absolutely *know* that the subconscious mind can turn mountains into molehills. The younger we are, the more likely this is to happen.

I absolutely *know* that it's not your tools or your techniques that makes healing possible; it's who you are as a healer.

I absolutely *know* that "convincing" a client isn't for show; it's for building a foundation for the faith required to *allow* healing to happen.

I absolutely *know* there *is* consciousness present inside the womb. There may not be what we call "thinking", but decisions are being made, just the same.

I absolutely *know* that the "first sense" is the "first imperative" for uncovering work. Sensing is subtler and goes beyond emotions and words.

I absolutely *know* how devastating the thought of separation feels. A child left alone in infancy can easily conclude that it will die. *That* is a biological conflict. (German New Medicine is really onto something here!)

I absolutely *know* that the session doesn't begin with the induction, and it doesn't end with emerging, which is why healing is about who you are, not just what you do.

I absolutely *know* that ongoing learning will help you to *be* a better healer because none of us has all the answers. (Fortunately, all we ever need are the questions!)

I absolutely *know* that if you're doing this work, you have been called to healing. But it's not a given. You must prepare yourself for the task. Know that you will make a positive difference in countless lives – many of which you will never meet.

> *The one who plants trees, knowing that he will never sit in their shade, has at least started to understand the meaning of life.*
>
> ~ Rabindranath Tagor

GLOSSARY OF TERMS

Abreaction: A physical movement or an emotional outburst as a reaction to a suggestion, while in the state of hypnosis. Some hypnotic abreactions are spontaneous, and others are created by the hypnotist. Hypnotic abreaction can be used to acquire greater depth, cause revivification, or remove repressed emotions.

Affect Bridge (AB): The technique whereby the client follows a feeling from the present to a past incident.[61]

Age progression (AP): Also known as future pacing, the client projects himself forward into the future. AP can be used to (a) test the client's expected results following hypnotherapeutic processing, (b) mentally rehearse future situations or event to experience successfully accomplishing a task, (c) to create future scenarios for the purpose of resource development, e.g. assertiveness training, (d) to see a desired outcome or the consequences of their current destructive behavior, e.g. High Road, Low Road, (e) compounding success by celebrating success in the future, (f) strategic planning by looking back from the future to see what concrete steps were taken to achieve success.

Age Regression (AR): The process of moving the client back in time from the present to a past incident to confront the cause of the presenting problem at its inception.

Anchoring: A neurolinguistic programming term for a natural process by which a conditioned response is formed. A memory, state, or behavior is associated (anchored) to a specific stimulus. Repeated stimuli then reinforce the association. The anchor (i.e. trigger or stimulus) can be physical (e.g. touch or sensation), visual (e.g. the color

---

[61] Developed by Joh G. Wakins

red), auditory (e.g. vocal tonality), verbal phrases (e.g. a word or phrase one says to oneself), as well as memories or emotional states (e.g. see a snake, feel fear). Also see Classical Conditioning.

Body Syndrome: a physical manifestation of an emotional trauma. When an emotion is held in or repressed instead of being processed and released, the emotion will express itself as a physical discomfort.

Chair Therapy (CT): This technique derives from the "empty chair technique" of Gestalt therapy, developed by Fritz Perls. Through this technique, the client is directed to place another person or part of himself (e.g. thought, feeling, symptom, aspect of a dream, etc.) in a chair across and several feet away from him. The client carries on a conversation by shifting back and forth between the 'other' and himself. This process allows the client to clarify his feelings and reactions to the other person and increase understanding. Understanding can then be used to facilitate forgiveness and behavioral change.

Classical Conditioning: A form of associative learning that was first demonstrated by Ivan Pavlov (1927) who trained dogs to salivate at the sound of a ringing bell. The conditioning process involves pairing a stimulus to a response. Through repetition the two become associated and the response becomes automatic (conditioned). E.g. fear conditioning. Also see anchoring.

Cognitive Bridge (CB): Rather than following a feeling, the client follows a thought back from the present to a past incident.

Conscious Mind (CM): In Sigmund Freud's psychoanalytic theory of personality, the conscious mind includes everything that is inside of our awareness. This is the aspect of our mental processing that we can think and talk about in a rational way. The conscious mind includes such things as the sensations, perceptions, memories, feelings and fantasies inside of our current awareness. Closely allied with the conscious mind is the preconscious, which includes the things that we are not thinking of at the moment but which we can easily draw into conscious awareness.

Convincer: Any method that provides the client with evidence and, therefore, firm his or her belief or a course of action. e.g. Eye Lock Test, Time Distortion Test, SUDS.

Core Beliefs: Beliefs that are installed prior to the establishment of the Critical Factor (usually before age 5). Example: "I'm unlovable." "I am stupid/ugly/incapable/etc."

Critical Function (CF): The semi-permeable barrier that sits between the conscious and subconscious mind which acts as a 'guardian at the gate' to protect our subconsciously held beliefs. It has the power to accept or reject suggestions. Suggestions that do not match existing programming automatically get rejected.

Deep Memory Process (DMP): A technique developed by Roger Woolger, PhD that combines Jungian analysis, psychodrama, and shamanic healing techniques to release ancestral or karmic issues, and to heal physical and emotional problems that are held in the body.

Direct Drive Technique (DDT): A compounding technique.[62] The law of compound suggestion states that once a suggestion has been accepted by the client's subconscious, it becomes easier for additional

---

[62] Developed by Gerald Kein, Omni-Hypnosis

suggestions to be accepted. With this process, the client repeats a single suggestion out loud with intention and enthusiasm (15 times or more).

Dark Force Entity (DFE): Also referred to as fallen angels, these spiritual parasites attach themselves to humans for their malicious purposes. They are hierarchical, clever, and are on a mission to gain power by destroying the light. They are often afraid of the light. DFE's have within them a spark of light but have been deceived into losing awareness of their true nature. The objective of Spirit Releasement Therapy (SRT) is to help them realize that they, themselves, are trapped so they can be release back to the light.[63]

Direct Suggestion (DS): Also known as authoritarian or paternal, this method was favored by Dave Elman. Suggestions are given in the form of instructions or commands, such as "*relax your eyelids to the point they just won't work*".

In contrast, indirect suggestion, or permissive/maternal, was the method favored by Milton Erickson. Indirect suggestions give the client the illusion of choice by deciding whether they will carry out the action requested by the hypnotist; for example, "*...and you might discover that your eyelids are becoming heavier.*" Another method that gives the illusion of choice is the double bind technique, which can be direct or indirect. For example: "*You can relax now, or you can relax later...whatever's best for you.*" This gives the client the illusion of choice, but presupposes that the client *will* relax, regardless of which option he chooses. This method is useful for analytical types who want to maintain control.

---

[63] To learn SRT, read Spirit Releasement Therapy by William J. Baldwin

Educational Pre-Talk: The process of educating a client in readiness for therapeutic hypnosis.

Ego States: Various aspects of the personality which formed in response to the client's life experiences. Healthy parts form in response to positive, loving, affirming relationships with role models. Wounded parts form in response to traumas, abuse, neglect, rejection, and enmeshing role models. These parts are stuck in the past where they continue to hold negative feelings and irrational beliefs which affect the client in the present. Also see Transactional Analysis.

Emotional Freedom Technique (EFT): Also known as 'tapping', the principle behind EFT is that negative emotions can cause disturbances in the body's energy field. EFT theory derives from similar principles behind those of acupuncture. EFT was originated by Gary Craig who studied TFT with Roger Callahan.

Energy Psychology: A group of meridian-based therapeutic methods which incorporate tapping, rubbing, or touching of acupressure points or chakras with or without the use of suggestions. Modalities include TFT, EFT, TAT, Seemorg Matrix Work, WHEE and others. (See MTT)

Finger Pinch Technique (FPT): The process whereby the rubbing or pinching of two fingers together is anchored to a specific response (e.g. feeling calm and relaxed)

Forgiveness of Others (FOO): The process of setting oneself free of the past by releasing anger, blame and condemnation toward an offender and finding some good in past transgressions. This serves to empower the forgiver to relinquish victim status and choose to take responsibility for their life and how they feel.

Forgiveness of Self (FOS): The process of releasing anger, blame and condemnation toward oneself by reframing past failings or transgressions as mistakes.

Future Pacing (FP): A.K.A. Age Progression, the process of guiding the client to imagine experiencing a future situation or event to test the results and reinforce change.

Grownup (GU): Adult consciousness of the client which can provide love, information, and guidance to the younger selves.

High Road, Low Road (HRLR): A 5-PATH adaptation of the Crossroads Patter. The client is guided to imagine him or herself standing at a crossroads. The past stretches out behind them, and the future lies before them along two distinct paths, one to the left and one to the right. The 'right' road is designated the High Road, while the road on the left is the Low Road. The client is then invited to travel down the Low Road to instill aversion to continuing their 'bad' behavior by looking at all the future negative consequences of continuing along this path. The client is then brought back to the crossroads to recognize they can still make the choice for change. They are then guided down the High Road to look at all the positive rewards of making this choice. The Crossroads Patter can also be used following successful clearing to allow the client to experience the road they are now on because of having made these positive changes. (i.e. future pacing)

Ignorant Spirit (IS): A.K.A. Earthbound Spirit, "hungry ghost," or "hitchhiker." According to spirit attachment theory, when a person dies and doesn't cross over into the light, he becomes earthbound and attaches to a living person. When death comes suddenly, the IS may be confused and not realize he is dead. If he is unwilling to let go of his physical existence he may avoid going into the light at the time of death. He may fear going to hell because of misdeeds during his life. Or, believing that nothing follows death, he may attempt to remain amongst the living. When an IS attaches to someone, it is generally out of ignorance rather than malice. He may become bound to someone with whom he has unfinished business. A grieving loved one may draw the IS to become attached to them in an attempt to comfort them. Substance abusers may attach to living users in an attempt to feed their addiction (hungry ghosts). A child may seek companionship with another child so as not to be alone.

Initial Sensitizing Event (ISE): A.K.A. "the seed-planting event" or "causal event." The first event which generated the perceptions underlying the client's presenting issue, usually occurring in childhood. The event is rarely known to the Conscious Mind. This event, while having an emotional impact at the time, may or may not have been traumatic. Each subsequent event which in some way resembles the first time then serves to re-stimulate the pattern established in the ISE, adding to its strength. Reframing the ISE will change the perceptions underlying the problem allowing a relieving of symptoms.

Inner Child (IC): The client at a younger age. Also referred to as the "Little One" or Child.

Intake Process: The preliminary interview in which a history of the client's presenting issue is taken.

Mental Rehearsal: the process of imagining or mentally practicing performing a task as opposed to actual practice.

Meridians: Biological energy lines in the body identified by Chinese Medicine thousands of years ago. Along these lines are sensitive points (acupuncture points) that can be stimulated to release blocks and stimulate the flow of bio-energies in the body for the purposes of healing.

Meridian Tapping Technique (MTT): MTT is the umbrella term for all techniques that utilize acupressure points to reduce or resolve negative emotions and the physical issues associated with them. Tapping practitioners use MTT to release blocks to the body's natural energy flow. Releasing the blocks allows the energy system to rebalance in the body-mind. Acupressure points are located where the meridian pathways are nearer to the skin's surface. Meridian tapping techniques address the energy system in the body by tapping or touching a number of these meridian points. MTT methods include Thought Field Therapy (TFT), Emotional Freedom Technique (EFT), Touch and Breath (TAB), Be Set Free Fast (BSFF), Thought Energy Synchronization Therapy (TEST), Negative Affect Erasing Method (NAEM) Individualized Energy Psychotherapy (IEP), Matrix Re-Imprinting, and others.

Muscle Response Test (MRT): A.K.A. muscle testing or kinesiology. A group of methods used to elicit unconscious (ideomotor) responses through the body. Developed by Dr. George Goodheart as a way to correct structural imbalances, MRT is used to retrieve information from the Subconscious through yes/no or true/false statements. There are various methods which include "the sway test," the Basic Arm Test, Hand Solo Method, Falling Log Method, Hole-In-One Method, and Linked Rings Method. MRT is used in the 'classic' approach to EFT. Dr. David Hawkins[64] utilized MRT to calibrate emotional energies.

---

[64] David Hawkins, Power vs Force

Parts: See Ego States. The primary Parts worked with in regression hypnotherapy sessions are the Inner Child, Adult Part, Parent Parts, and Offender.

Parts Therapy (PT): A.K.A. Ego State Therapy, Subpersonality Work, Parts Mediation Therapy. This method has its roots in Gestalt Therapy. Conflicting parts are identified and then communicated with to bring about resolution. Parts Therapy was pioneered by [Charles Tebbetts](). His work is carried out today by C. Roy Hunter.

Past Life Regression (PLR): Regression to an event in a previous incarnation. The belief in past lives is common to many spiritual systems, including early Christianity, which believe in the eternal nature of the soul which reincarnates. The Yoga Sutras of Patanjali discuss the concept of karma. Karma is essentially the concept of free will; humans have free will to choose good or evil and then experience the consequences of their choices. The soul is believed to be burdened with an accumulation of impressions which are carried over from previous lives.

Progressive Relaxation (PR): Progressive Relaxation generally applies to a relaxation induction. The client is instructed to focus inside the body and, starting at either the top of the head or the feet, imagine relaxing various muscles in a sequential manner. Originally known as Progressive muscle relaxation (PMR), this technique was developed by Edmund Jacobson in the early 1920s as a means of relieving anxiety. Jacobson believed that since muscle tension accompanies anxiety, one can reduce anxiety by relaxing the muscular tension. By sequentially tensing and relaxing muscles in the legs, abdomen, chest, arms and face, anxiety is, therefore, systematically reduced. Jacobson discovered that this technique is also effective with ulcers, insomnia, and hypertension.

Set-up Statement: A precise statement used to focus the mind on the thoughts, feelings and memories associated with an issue prior to a round of releasing.

Somatic Bridge: Rather than following a feeling or a thought, the client focuses on a physical sensation and follows it back from the present to a past incident.

Somnambulism: Considered a 'working depth' of hypnosis for regression work. This level is easy to test for and provides a very clear and measurable result. Tests include Numbers Challenge (losing the numbers), Eye Fractionation Test, Pinch Test for analgesia, hallucination through suggestion.

Spirit Releasement Therapy (SRT): Sometimes referred to as "a clinical approach to de-possession", SRT was developed by the late Dr. William Baldwin.

Subconscious Mind (SCM/SM): A.K.A. the Feeling Mind. The part of the mind that is below the threshold of consciousness. The SCM is responsible for feelings, intuition, imagination, and holds all the memories. It is the seat of our emotions and is the driving force of our being.

Subjective Unit of Distress Scale (SUDS): Also known as 'Subjective Units of Disturbance Scale'. The client assesses their level of discomfort using an intensity scale, usually 0 to 10 where 10 is "the worst it has ever been" and 0 is zero distress or "peaceful and comfortable." This self-assessment tool guides the Hypnotherapist while providing the client with convincing evidence of improvement. The SUDS can be used prior to releasing as well as retroactively.

Subsequent Sensitizing Event (SSE): Events subsequent to the ISE which reinforce the causal event generating a pattern of behavior and/or survival. When life events match the ISE, the pattern of behavior/survival is reinforced and internal stress increases.

Symptom Producing Event (SPE): The most recently occurring SSE where the underlying problem began to express as symptoms. e.g. client took up smoking or overeating, the rash appeared, etc.

Transactional Analysis (TA): Eric Berne's ego states[65]; Parent, Adult and Child are the three basic 'parts' worked with during regression. TA explains why people respond the way they do to various situations (i.e. behavioral patterns).

Unconscious Mind (UCM): A.K.A. Body Mind. The deepest stratum of the subconscious mind is responsible for automatic body functions such as heart rate, respiration, digestion, elimination, perspiration, etc.

Ultra-Depth (UD): A.K.A. The Sichort State. To achieve this profound depth of consciousness and awareness, the individual must be conditioned to first achieve profound Somnambulism. The individual must then be conditioned to the Esdaile State (coma state) and be tested by catatonic responses. Finally, the individual must achieve the Sichort State where it is possible to instantly induce either analgesia, local or general anesthetic suitable for surgery. Regressions in the Sichort State bring forth the actual past personality. In most

---

[65] Parts or subpersonalities

cases, the subject will have no conscious recall. This is the same state achieved by Edgar Cayce for the purpose of trance channeling. The only level of depth below the Sichort State is natural deep sleep. James Ramey continues the work of Walter Sichort.

Ultra-Height (UH): A method created by Gerald F. Kein which allows the client to reach expanded levels of awareness where he or she can readily obtain knowledge and insight to their physical, mental and/or emotional problems. To achieve this state, the client is first guided into a state of somnambulism. S/he is then guided deeper into the Esdaile State (coma state). Once the Esdaile State is achieved, the client is guided to allow the mind to float free of the body and drift up to increasingly higher planes of consciousness. This heightened state of awareness and mental clarity can be used to identify the root cause of a problem as well as the solution, seek guidance, access knowledge, and achieve healing.

The Devil's Therapy Series

Book 1: The Devil's Therapy: *Hypnosis Practitioner's Essential Guide to Effective Regression Hypnotherapy*

Book 2: Ditch the Pitch: *Simple Proven Client Attraction Strategies for Hypnosis Practitioners Who Don't Love Digital Marketing*

Book 3: Ditch the Script: *Get Everything You Need from the Client for Successful Hypnotherapy and Set Up to Wrap Up with Results*

Book 4: Radical Healing: *Hypnosis Practitioner's Guide to Harnessing the Healing Power of the Educational Pretalk*

Book 5: The Devil's Little Black Book: *Regression Hypnotherapist's Troubleshooting Guide with Tips, Tricks & Even Scripts to Tweak Your Therapeutic Technique*

Book 6: The Dream Healing Practitioner Guidebook: *A Healer's Guide to Uncovering the Secret Messages of Your Dreams*

Book 7: Ready for Regression: *Hypnosis Practitioner's Guide to Preparing Clients for Effective Regression Hypnotherapy*

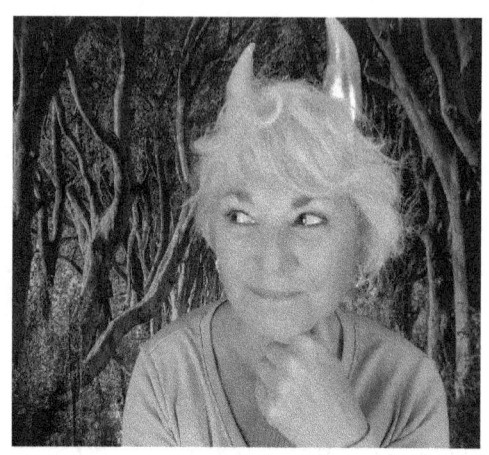

Wendie Webber

With over thirty years of experience as a healing practitioner, Wendie brings a broad range of skills to her unique approach to Regression to Cause hypnosis.

She is an Omni-Hypnosis graduate, 5-Path practitioner, Transactional hypnotherapist, Alchemical hypnotherapist, Satir Transformational Systemic therapist, and Regression Hypnotherapy Boot Camp participant.

Before hypnosis, Wendie owned a self-help bookstore where she explored spirituality, psychology, and energy-based healing.

Wendie is the recipient of the 2006 5-PATH Leadership Award and the 2019 Gerald F. Kein OMNI Award for Excellence in Hypnotism.

She enjoys an eclectic lifestyle on Vancouver Island, British Columbia, Canada, surrounded by nature, oracles, and cats.

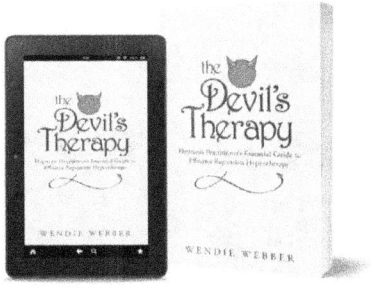

The Devil's Therapy: *Hypnosis Practitioner's Essential Guide to Effective Regression Hypnotherapy.* Discover how a 200-year-old fairy tale reveals a complete system for facilitating effective regression hypnotherapy. Learn the "Why" behind the "How-To" of regression to cause hypnosis. Turn your hypnosis sessions into healing programs and get results that last. This practical guidebook gives you a step-by-step map you can use to facilitate successful regression therapy. It's much simpler than you might imagine.

This is absolutely amazing work. It's so clear and precise, just like a laser. It leaves no doubts about what to do, how to do it, and the best part: Why to do it!! - **Zoran Pavlovic, Belgrade, Serbia**

The Devil's Therapy provides a simple three-phase, seven-step protocol for facilitating regression to cause therapeutic hypnosis. The first phase is comprised of three steps which effectively set up for a multi-session healing program. The second phase is comprised of two steps which make up the core work of regression to cause and inner child work. The third phase involves the final two steps of testing/integrating all changes followed by the forgiveness work.

Available on Amazon in English, German, and French versions.

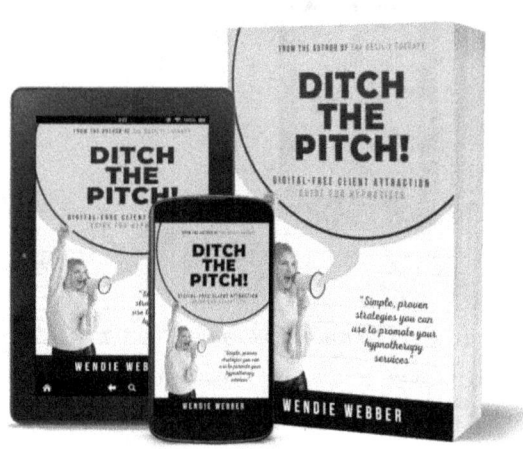

Ditch the Pitch! Digital Free Client Attraction Guide for Hypnotists is a beginner's guide to marketing yourself and your services *without* having to do that dreaded sales pitch, figure out how to game the algorithms on social media, or stay on top of SEO. This is an old-school, hands-on approach for healers who want to take care of business by connecting with real people who truly need your help. That's it.

> *"I've paid a lot of money for business courses and never completed them. I felt overwhelmed and lost in all the content. This course was easy, simple to follow, and taught me so much. I feel confident and ready to change my current system and start implementing what I've learned in my own practice".* – **Nicole D**

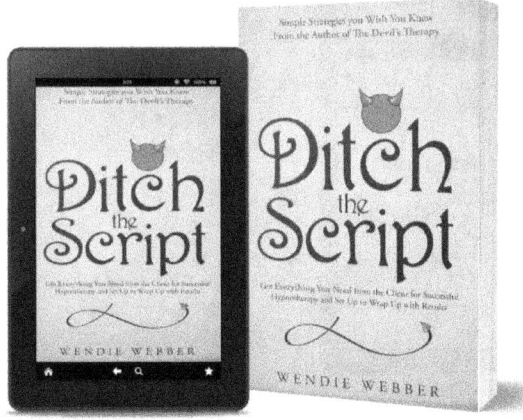

Ditch the Script: *Get Everything You Need from the Client for Successful Hypnotherapy and Set Up to Wrap Up with Results.* Your success is always going to be in your set up. Ditch the Script reveals simple strategies you can use right away to break free of 'scriptnotism' and start facilitating client-centered regression to cause therapeutic hypnosis. Learn how to qualify your clients, conduct the strategic intake process, and more.

> *I read the first chapter before bed. Wow! Really good! Can't wait to absorb this book!! I didn't think anything could top the first book. After reading one chapter of this second book. I was clearly wrong!* – **Michael Madden, USA**

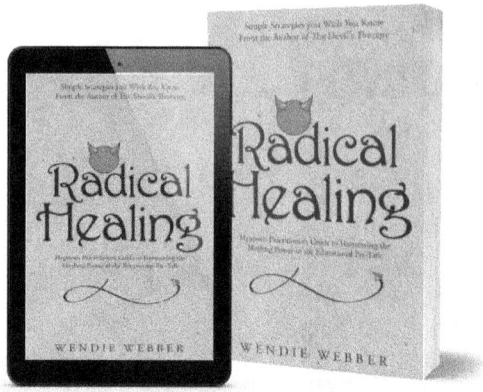

Radical Healing: *Hypnosis Practitioner's Guide to Harnessing the Healing Power of the Educational Pretalk.* Learn how to prepare your clients for a body-centered approach to healing the mind. Discover how every phase of the healing process involves a contract – from the initial call with a prospective client, to the first session, for the hypnosis, and for regression.

> *Wendie's lessons have been invaluable in helping me to understand the subconscious mind and I feel like I really get it now. I used what I learned right away to great effect with my clients, and it has taken my practice to a whole new level of learning. My clients are seeing results faster! The insights and healing just come more naturally, now – it just seems to flow easily.* – **Craig Homonnay, Australia**

> **, USA**

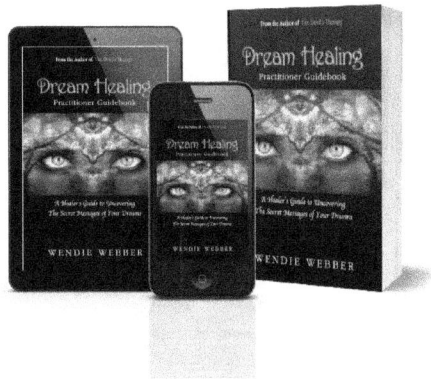

Dream Healing Practitioner Guidebook: *A Healer's Guide to Uncovering the Secret Messages of Your Dreams*. Learn deceptively simple techniques you can use – yourself and with others – to uncover the meaning of your dreams. If you're a healing practitioner, *Dream Healing* gives you an insight therapy you can offer to clients. *Dream Healing* can help you to develop valuable skills that can support you in your healing sessions with clients. Working with your own dreams can help you to develop intuition while bringing balance and harmony to your mind-body system.

Makes Things So Simple

I have thoroughly loved working with dream healing tools. Wendie makes things so simple and easy that learning new skills such as dream healing become easy to apply and implement from the start. I have absolutely loved uncovering my dream meanings and then putting what I've learnt into action because understanding a dream is not enough; it also needs some change/action for resolution to happen. It's been such an interesting and fun experience. Thank you, so much! – **Nicole Dodd, UK**

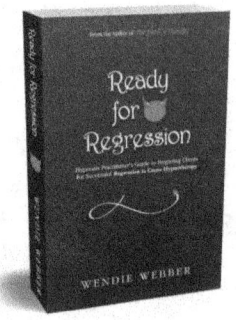

Ready for Regression: *Hypnosis Practitioner's Guide to Preparing Clients for Effective Regression Hypnotherapy.* The Ready for Regression First Session System is based on a five-star rated course. Gain the confidence you need to guide your clients through the multiple healing processes of Regression to cause therapeutic hypnosis.

> *IT WORKS!!!! I just finished a NEW session with a NEW client located in Asia. I had my semi-completed session manual with me that I put together based on your training course and . . . wow. It works. Confidence was back. Client felt great. Deep trance. I could go on forever. In short - thank you, Wendie. I put your course and method to real life and IT WORKS!!!!!! It works!!!! A huge suffocating hug to you!!! Thank you!!! And I didn't even complete all the courses yet!!!*
>
> *~ Jo Nontakorn*

Get clear. Get confident

www.ingramcontent.com/pod-product-compliance
Lightning Source LLC
Chambersburg PA
CBHW070522010526
44118CB00012B/1052